OTA Exam Review Manual

Second Edition

OTA Exam Review Manual

Second Edition

Karen Sladyk, PhD, OTR/L, FAOTA
Bay Path College
Longmeadow, Massachusetts

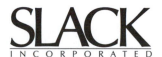

SLACK
INCORPORATED

an innovative information, education, and management company
6900 Grove Road • Thorofare, NJ 08086

Copyright © 2005 by SLACK Incorporated

ISBN 10: 1-55642-701-8
ISBN 13: 9781556427015

The author, editor, and publisher cannot accept responsibility for errors or exclusions or for the outcome of the application of the material presented herein. There is no expressed or implied warranty of this book or information imparted by it.

The work SLACK publishes is peer reviewed. Prior to publication, recognized leaders in the field, educators, and clinicians provide important feedback on the concepts and content that we publish. We welcome feedback on this work.

The material in this book has been compiled to help the student review and prepare for the certification exam. The author and the publisher are not responsible for errors or omissions, or for the consequences from application of the book, and makes no warranty, expressed or implied, in regard to the contents of the book.

Several questions in this exam guide involve information about medications commonly taken by occupational therapy consumers. Copyright information is provided below and cited from *The physician's desk reference* (53rd ed.). (1999). Montvale, NJ: Medical Economics Company. The following medications are generic and may be produced by one or more pharmaceutical companies: imipramine, levodopa, heparin, baclofen, and clonidine. The following brand name products are trademarked by the following companies: **Alka-Seltzer**, Bayer Corporation, Morristown, NJ; **Dantrium**, Procter & Gamble Pharmaceuticals, Cincinnati, OH; **Prozac**, Dista Products/Eli Lilly and Company, Indianapolis, IN; **Ridaura**, Connetics Corporation, Palo Alto, CA; **Ritalin**, Novartis Pharmaceuticals, Basel, Switzerland; **Thorazine**, SmithKline Beecham Pharmaceuticals, Philadelphia, PA; **Tylenol**, McNeil Consumer Products, Fort Washington, PA; and **Valium**, Roche Pharmaceuticals, Manati, PR.

Sladyk, Karen, 1958-
 OTA exam review manual / Karen Sladyk.-- 2nd ed.
   p. ; cm.
 Includes bibliographical references and index.
 ISBN-10: 1-55642-701-8 (pbk.)
 ISBN-13: 978-1-55642-701-5 (pbk.)
 1. Occupational therapy--Examinations, questions, etc. 2. Occupational therapy--Outlines, syllabi, etc. 3. Occupational therapy assistants.
 [DNLM: 1. Occupational Therapy--Examination Questions. WB 18.2 S631o 2005] I. Title.

RM735.32.S536 2005
615.8'515'076--dc22

                                        2004029297

Printed in the United States of America.
Published by: SLACK Incorporated
                          6900 Grove Road
                          Thorofare, NJ 08086-9447 USA
                          Telephone: 856-848-1000
                          Fax: 856-853-5991
                          www.slackbooks.com

Contact SLACK Incorporated for more information about other books in this field or about the availability of our books from distributors outside the United States.

Authorization to photocopy items for internal or personal use, or the internal or personal use of specific clients, is granted by SLACK Incorporated, provided that the appropriate fee is paid directly to Copyright Clearance Center, 222 Rosewood Drive, Danvers, MA 01923 USA, 978-750-8400. Prior to photocopying items for educational classroom use, please contact the CCC at the address above. Please reference Account Number 9106324 for SLACK Incorporated's Professional Book Division.

For further information on CCC, check CCC Online at the following address: http://www.copyright.com.

Last digit is print number: 10 9 8 7 6 5 4 3 2 1

DEDICATION

To every occupational therapy assistant student and the teachers
and clinicians who educate them.

Contents

Section I. Getting Ready

Karen Sladyk, PhD, OTR, FAOTA and Lori Vaughn, OTR/L

Section II. Study Techniques

Lori S. Gilmore, MS, CSE

Section III. Study Questions

Section IV. Life After the Exam

Appendices

About the Authors

Dr. Karen Sladyk has a Bachelor of Science in Occupational Therapy from Eastern Michigan University, Ypsilanti, MI; a Master of Science in Community Health Education from Southern Connecticut State University, New Haven, CT; and a PhD in Adult and Vocational Education from the University of Connecticut, Storrs, CT. She is currently Professor and Chair of Occupational Therapy at Bay Path College in Longmeadow, MA. Her interests include clinical reasoning and professional development of students. She is author/editor of *OT/OTA Study Cards in a Box* and *OT Student Primer* and coauthor/coeditor of *OT Exam Review Manual, Third Edition* and *Ryan's Occupational Therapy Assistant, Third Edition*. She lives in a small house in historical Tolland, CT, with two cats and enjoys quilt making in her free time.

Lori S. Gilmore has a Bachelor of Science in Social Work from Southern Connecticut State University, a teaching certificate in special education, a Master of Science in Language Arts from Central Connecticut State University, New Britain, CT, and a sixth-year in learning disabilities from the University of Connecticut. When she is not busy with work, she is active in school and community projects with her new family including her three sons, Brent, Seth, and Blake. Lori also teaches and enjoys quilt making, but is much different from her sister Karen in that she only has one cat.

The OT and OTA students of the Bay Path College Class of 2001 participated in a collaborative project as part of their management class. This project had teams of OT and OTA students working together to develop study question content. Dr. Karen Sladyk proudly lists their names here:

OT students:
Diane Archambault, COTA
Susan Choronzy
Laurie DiNicola-Landry
Sarah Goddard
Diane Kabaniuk
Emilie Pessagno
Barbara Vagen Saladin, COTA
Nikki Segal
Shana Teed
Jennifer Zawistowski-Sweetland

OTA students:
Alicia Cavanagh
Guinevere Gonyea
Amy Kingsbury
Laura Mancuso
Sarah Smith
Candace White
Tracy Williams

In this new edition, Lori Vaughn, OT/R, adds her voice to the study process in preparing for the NBCOT exam.

PREFACE

Each year as I get to know more occupational therapy students, I am amazed at the hard work they put forth in becoming practitioners. I am lucky to teach at a college that offers a Master of Science in Occupational Therapy and formerly an Associate of Science in Occupational Therapy Assisting. I teach at a small college, where I can get to know all the OT and OTA students. I am also lucky that I work with some of the best OT faculty around—faculty that say "okay" when I suggested that we combine the two programs for a collaborative project and have the students work together to develop some of the study questions in this book.

With the input of students and several professionals, I have developed a new study guide to prepare for the NBCOT exam. Some may wonder why I wrote another exam review guide when there are already several excellent "official" and "unofficial" study guides on the market. I believed that I could contribute to the success of students by providing "a just right challenge" study guide. One with a reasonable amount of questions, not too many to overwhelm or be superficial, and not too little to leave you looking for more. This study guide, like its sister *OT Exam Review Manual, Fourth Edition*, provides supportive information that assists students in the studying process.

This book provides facts that you need to know but also includes celebrations of the information you already know. When possible, a lighter, humorous side of information sharing is used. You may notice that the chapter on studying for the exam is written by my sister. She wrote a similar chapter for the *OT Exam Review Manual, Fourth Edition* using humor to address a subject you know all too well. The original *OT Exam Review Manual* had two of my favorite colleagues from the professional degree program at Quinnipiac University. Even though I no longer work with them day-to-day and they did not participate in this OTA version, I want to thank Roseanna Tufano and Signian McGeary for helping me become a better writer and a better teacher. Special thanks to Robin Clark, who did an outstanding job editing the text for me. As always, thanks to Amy Drummond, Rob Smentek, and all my friends at SLACK Incorporated for making me look so good.

This exam review manual is designed to help the OTA student move from fieldwork to the NBCOT exam. The first chapters provide scheduling and studying tips, content review outlines, and fieldwork review examples. The study questions are designed to help you study—not necessarily "practice"—for the exam. To that degree, a wide variety of questions, both simple and complex, are included in this book. Answers explain why one choice is correct and why the others are incorrect. There is even a chapter on how to handle not passing the exam the first time. In addition, a companion Web site has been created with domain-style study questions to accompany the book. The testing site has a 4-hour time limit to resemble the actual certification exam as closely as possible. You have the option of restarting the test three times before it goes into a review-only mode. You may also exit the test at any time and restart it to continue where you left off, as long as you have not exceeded the 4-hour time limit. The Web site is a first for this book and is an "added value" to the study process as the exam moves to computerized format.

I would love to hear how you found this manual in your studying. You can write to me care of SLACK Incorporated, 6900 Grove Road, Thorofare, NJ 08086. All the best on your new career. I am sure you will enjoy your new path as much as I have.

Karen Sladyk, PhD, OTR/L, FAOTA

SECTION I
Getting Ready

Chapter One

The Exam Process

Karen Sladyk, PhD, OTR/L, FAOTA, and Lori Vaughn, OTR/L

WHAT TO DO FIRST

Many students preparing for the OTA exam ask the question, "What should I do first?" The answer is, "It depends." This study guide includes information for every type of person. Where you start depends on how much time you have left to study and who you are. In an attempt to give you some structure, let's first look at how much time you have between opening this book for the first time and the next certification exam. The student should check the National Board for Certification in Occupational Therapy's (NBCOT) Web site (www.nbcot.org) on a regular basis to receive up-to-the-minute information. As for studying, calculate the time you have until the next exam and check the table below for a suggestion of what to do next.

WHAT TO DO FIRST	
Time left until next exam:	*Start your reading here:*
6 or more months	Good for you! You have plenty of time to study. Read the entire study guide. Study 1 to 2 hours per week initially.
4 to 5 months	You planned well. Read the entire study guide. Begin with 3 to 4 hours per week.
2 to 3 months	No need to panic—you have some time, but you must be efficient. Read the entire study guide except for the questions this week. Aim for an hour per day until the study questions are complete, then adjust your study time from there.
About 1 month	Time to get serious. Read the entire study guide this week. Aim for at least 1 to 2 hours per day until it is complete. Begin your study plan developed in Chapter Two.
3 weeks 100	Skip Chapters One and Seven for now. Begin Chapter Two. Then try at least questions in Chapter Six. Adjust your study plan from there.
2 weeks	Move right to Chapter Six and complete. Skim Chapters Two, Four, and Five. Review Chapter Three. Develop a study plan from there.
1 week or less	Move right to Chapter Six and complete. Skim Chapter Four for test-taking suggestions. Review Chapter Three. Develop a study plan from there.
If you are already an OTA and are using this book for review	If taking the exam, begin with Chapters Five and Six. Skim Chapters Two and Three. If not taking the exam but doing a review, complete Chapters Five and Six and review Chapter Three.

Assuming you have at least 40 hours of study time ahead of you, the entire study guide is within your reach. A good place to start is right here. A little history about the certification process will give you a better understanding of the exam.

CERTIFICATION PROCESS

The NBCOT is a private nonprofit agency responsible for the development and administration of the certification exam for OTs and OTAs. Management of each exam requires development of high standards to protect and serve the public. This assures quality occupational therapy personnel are entering the profession. NBCOT meets the challenge by developing policies and working closely with the development committee and test and measurement experts to assure quality. Although certification of an OTA may not be required by some work sites, most governmental, regulatory, insurance, and other agencies use NBCOT examinations as a credentialing standard. Many states' licensing boards require passing the certification exam as the minimum standard for employment.

OTA Examination Question Development

The questions on the OTA certification exam are based on a survey conducted of practitioners and educators to establish the knowledge of entry-level clinicians. The study focused on the skills needed by a new graduate to successfully practice occupational therapy. The study results are used by the Certification Examination Development Committee (CEDC) to develop new exam questions.

Expert OTs and OTAs from a variety of work settings across the country make up the NBCOT's CEDC. The members of this committee are trained in item writing and develop exam questions specific to their content area. All items are rigorously reviewed by the CEDC before appearing as examination questions. Item writers use AOTA's *The Practice Framework* for terminology. This publication is available in the *American Journal of Occupational Therapy*, November/December, 2002 or by calling AOTA at (301) 652-2682 (1-800-SAY-AOTA if you are a student member).

OTA Examination Administration

The NBCOT contracts with a professional testing company to assure high standards of reliability and validity in test development and administration. The professional testing agency is responsible for administering and scoring the exam, as well as reporting the results to the candidate. Beginning in September 2001, NBCOT contracted community learning centers to administer the computerized version.

Each OTA certification exam is a unique combination of exam items pulled from a data bank of possible questions. The data banks for OTAs and OTs are kept separate, and the questions are never used in both examinations. NBCOT provides a list of content areas and the percentage of weight for each area to the test taker prior to the exam. This outline assures consistency between the tests over time.

Application for the OTA Examination

It is the student's responsibility to initiate the application process to take the OTA exam. Your program director can help you with this process. Students in their last year of school should check NBCOT's Web site (www.nbcot.org) on a regular basis to stay up-to-date with the application process. Candidates can now apply for the exam either online or by using traditional mail applications. The nice things about applying online is that the application will warn you if you left a line blank, and online applications are less expensive. Errors on the written application are not returned but held until the exam. NBCOT has a candidate handbook that provides detailed information on the application process. Be sure to follow all rules completely and carefully, especially where fees are concerned.

OTA Examination Structure

Each exam has 200 multiple-choice questions. Each question will have four possible choices labeled A, B, C, and D. There are no "all of the above," "except," or combination choices on the OTA exam. The penalty for leaving an answer blank is the same as an incorrect answer, so be sure to type your best guess for all items. The computerized test will only accept one answer. Even if you are unsure of an answer, use your best guess in order to avoid an empty or wrong answer.

After flawed pilot questions are removed, criterion-referenced scoring will be used to calculate the passing score. This means that those people above the criterion score will pass the certification examination and those below will not. Your score is not compared to other people who took the exam but simply compared to the minimum passing level to be an entry-level occupational therapy assistant. Generally, the pass rate has been about 80%.

Test takers who need special accommodations due to a disability (such as visual, hearing, health, or orthopedic impairment; or learning, emotional, or multiple disabilities) will be provided with services as outlined in the Americans with Disabilities Act. Information on special accommodations is located in the candidate's handbook from NBCOT. It is important that you provide the documentation necessary and follow the specific process in the handbook. Students with documented disabilities should begin the application process early to allow time to gather all needed material.

OTA EXAMINATION STRUCTURE

The "New" NBCOT Exam

Beginning in March 2000, NBCOT developed a new style of certification exam to reflect the most recent professional practice survey completed in 2003. This section of the book will look at the facts about the "new" exam.

Much of the new exam structure remains unchanged. The exam still consists of 200 multiple-choice questions with four possible answers. The candidates still have 4 hours to answer their questions on a computer. The questions are still entry-level occupational therapy assisting practice questions from a variety of practice areas. So what's the difference? The difference is how the questions are developed and classified.

Domain, Tasks, Knowledge

The most recent practice analysis survey looked at what OTAs need to know to practice occupational therapy. NBCOT developed a new blue print in 2004 based on the practice analysis of 2003. The new structure of the exam is based on three components of a new practitioner's work - domains, tasks, and knowledge. Although no major changes were the result of this new blueprint, NBCOT has used new language that better fits what the practice setting is using. Under NBCOT's 2004 blueprint, domains include:

- Evaluation
- Developing treatment plans
- Implementing meaningful treatment approaches
- Addressing population needs
- Managing OT services

Domains continue to be the foundation of the exam and implementing meaningful interventions continues to be the area of heaviest test questions. *Tasks* are described as what practitioners do and *knowledge* is defined as what practitioners need to know to perform tasks. Under the old blueprint, these two areas were described as content. So why is this language change so important to the person studying for the exam? Because it reinforces that your study approach must be holistic and not just focused on treatment from a pathology point of view. That said, you must also have a firm knowledge base of foundations, pathology, and management issues. The blueprint, is just that, a plan or guide for NBCOT to outline questions that are as diverse as the practice of occupational therapy.

Using the domain, task, knowledge blueprint, consider the following case: A person with a vestibular disorder of disequilibrium due to aging is referred to occupational therapy. She is complaining that balance problems interfere with her activities.

For domain issues, you must think about evaluation, treatment, and issues of importance to this population. For task issues, you must think about what OT practitioners do with clients such as this. For knowledge issues, you must think about pathology and foundations of meaningful activities. Note how tasks and knowledge help form the domain and how the 3 categories are all interlinked. This is the holistic nature of the exam questions.

Knowledge needed for the specific case of vestibular disorder of disequilibrium due to aging includes:
- There is likely loss of cells in the peripheral labyrinth as well as the CNS
- This likely developed over time
- There is likely loss of sensation in the foot, perhaps diabetes
- There is likely proprioception issues.

Tasks common for this specific case of vestibular disorder of disequilibrium due to aging includes:
- Activities must be graded
- Transfers from sitting to standing is likely an issue, especially the bathtub
- Patient education

A domain-based question that utilizes knowledge and tasks would look like this: A person with a vestibular disorder of disequilibrium due to aging is referred to occupational therapy. She is complaining that balance interferes with her socializing even in her house because she cannot wash and dress herself. What is the first issue for the OTA to address?

A. Finding ways for her to socialize using the phone

B. Addressing safety in the bathtub

C. Improving balance during dressing

D. Developing a graded exercise program to improve balance

The best answer is B. All the options, finding activities that are meaningful to this client, are appropriate treatment but the first issue is always safety. As a person with this condition may have sensation issues, especially if diabetes is present, bathtub mobility becomes a safety issue immediately.

There are no questions on the NBCOT exam that ask task or knowledge questions. An example of a task questions would be: How do OTAs adapt a bathroom? An example of a knowledge question would be: What inner ear cells are likely lost in aging? Since this type of question is never asked on the NBCOT exam, why include these in this study manual?

Mixed Domain, Task, and Knowledge Questions as Study Questions

This exam manual uses all three types of questions as a way to prepare you for the NBCOT exam. The questions in this book are designed as study tools, not real practice questions. On a rare occasion, we received feedback that our questions "were not like the real test." This test taker was right, these questions are designed to help you study all the material necessary to be confident in your answers on the NBCOT exam. Simply practicing real questions will only give you a pass/fail score, not prepare you to think about the questions. This goes back to the earlier comment about preparing for the NBCOT from a holistic approach including using a variety of study ideas.

WHEN TWO SOURCES DISAGREE

A student wrote us once asking for our opinion about a specific question, where our information disagreed with the information she had obtained from another resource. We were happy to comment on this because in an exciting and always changing profession like occupational therapy, there are times when professionals disagree about an issue. Our questions are study questions, designed to help you study for the exam. Because the questions are not exam questions, you may find a question where the answer disagrees with something you learned somewhere else. In the NBCOT exam, numerous people review each question. Remember that NBCOT also removes any question from the exam after it has been administered if the question is found to be faulty. Always trust your best judgment in making your final choice.

STUDYING IDEAS

Now that you understand NBCOT and the certification process, it is time to make your study plan. Chapter Two of this book covers your personal study plan in great detail; however, let us briefly look at some studying ideas you may find helpful.

Study groups: Studying a large amount of material with a group of people can be easier and more efficient. However, not all study groups are effective. You may have experienced a group project in school where one or more participants did not do their fair share. This often leads to resentment and hurt feelings. If you plan to form a study group, ask people you know will actively participate. If you are asked to join a study group, be sure you have a clear understanding of the group's goals, expectations, and work load. In any case, be sure to allow some time at the beginning of the first session to allow everyone an opportunity to share goals and expectations. If someone feels she cannot participate, allow her to decline with dignity.

Exam review conferences: Many occupational therapy schools offer a 1- or 2-day conference to review for the exam. You can call AOTA if you are a member or area occupational therapy schools to see if they are hosting a review conference.

Lecture notes: Even though you may have had one class that you did not like, the faculty at your school has provided you with a global education in occupational therapy assisting. AOTA requires all occupational therapy programs to meet minimum standards to receive or maintain the school's accreditation. Your occupational therapy program has met the standard regulations. This means that your classes provided you with at least the minimum information needed to pass the exam and become a practicing OTA. With all of that said, you should have everything you need to know about occupational therapy written down in your class lecture notes. Reviewing your notes is one of the most effective ways to study for the certification exam.

Textbooks: It would be impossible (and we do not recommend) that you try to reread your textbooks from cover to cover. Even if you did not sell them back to the bookstore for some extra cash, reading your textbooks in their entirety is not an effective use of study time.

It is appropriate to read your textbooks in the areas in which you are weak. We recommend that you read only the textbook sections in which you need detailed review. Use your notes from class to provide a basic study outline and refer to the textbooks for more detail. Be sure to save your textbooks for your professional needs after the exam.

NBCOT practice exam: For an additional charge, NBCOT offers a practice test given by computer online. The test is made up of sample questions scored by computer and a summary of your scores is provided. See the application to sign up for this practice test.

We would also like to call your attention to the appendices of this book, which provide information that you may find helpful as you study for the exam. In Appendix A, you will find a list of suggested occupational therapy references. Do not worry if you have never had a particular textbook in your classes. The suggestions are comprehensive to provide broad coverage of the material on the exam; however, your faculty has chosen an excellent blend of textbooks for you. In addition to the reference list, we have provided a list of abbreviations in Appendix B that you may find helpful as you study. All of this information is designed to help you get ready for the "big day."

EXAM DAY

The day of the exam will be filled with much nervous energy. It is best to plan ahead to enhance the chances of a smooth day. Old advice of a good night's sleep and eating well before any test is especially true for taking the "big" exam. You may want to try a dry run to the test site prior to exam day if you are unfamiliar with the location. If you are traveling on an exam day that might have bad weather, listen to the weather report and allow extra time to get to the exam site if needed. If you are driving, fill the gas tank the day before the exam.

Wear comfortable clothes but keep in mind the season and weather. Layered clothing will allow you to adjust your clothing if the room is too warm or cool. If your hair is long, tie it back, but avoid wearing a baseball cap or other type of hat that blocks your face from the exam proctors.

Have a bag ready to take with you as you leave for the test site. Include the following items in your bag:
- Map and phone number to the test site if you are unfamiliar with the location
- A cell phone or change for a pay phone to call for directions or help if needed
- A watch
- Photo identification
- Tissues are provided at the test site, but you may want to bring your own earplugs
- A snack high in complex carbohydrates (e.g., whole-grain bagel) for long-term thinking power; eat before entering the testing room, as food is not allowed during the exam
- Chewing gum, if needed
- Reading glasses, if you use them
- Your admission paperwork
- A pencil if you want to use scratch paper

Once you arrive at the test site, get in line to register. You may want to use the restroom while waiting to enter the exam room. If you are anxious, avoid talking to people who will make you feel more nervous. Find a quiet space to relax. Do not study or review notes. This is the time to focus on relaxing.

A NEW OT'S VOICE

In this edition of the book, we have provided feedback from a new OT who recently completed the study process for the new NBCOT exam. Here is her story to share. We hope you enjoy her insights.

From the Desk of Lori Vaughn, OTR/L

In occupational therapy, there is nothing more exhilarating, or terrifying, than completing the academic requirements and fieldwork affiliations and walking toward the podium to accept your diploma at graduation. Exhilarating because you are taking the first steps toward the rest of your life. Terrifying because you are taking the first steps toward the rest of your life. Before the calligrapher's ink has dried on your diploma, the realization hits that the journey is only half over, and you must now prepare for the NBCOT registration exam.

Undertaking preparations to study is no easy task. The volumes of information that you accumulated while in school and during fieldwork can seem like an incredible, insurmountable mountain. Each day you avoid the mountain, which in actuality is the closed door behind which you have hidden all of your school "stuff." Perhaps you are hoping it will go away, thinking that if you don't look at it, it doesn't exist. Or, maybe you just cannot get over that nausea that you feel every time you think about taking the exam. "I just need a break," I would tell myself. "I'm not ready yet," was another excuse. I was just overwhelmed.

One day I received an information letter regarding repayment of my student loans. This was my wake-up call, and I realized that I could no longer continue with my excuses. My future was coming whether I was ready or not. I knew that there was only one way for me to buckle down, and that was to bite the bullet and schedule a date for the exam.

Once I had a date scheduled, I was like a woman possessed. Typically, I am an organization freak (I have been called the queen of color coding), which I believe was ultimately the key to my success. Everyone has his or her own study strategies, and the ones I describe may not be for everyone, but they worked for me. First, I bravely repeated the phrase that became my mantra throughout this experience, "You can do it... You can do it..." and opened that dreaded door separating me from the rest of my life. I began organizing the class notes and information that were beginning to gather dust, much like my brain. As the piles of information grew, I began to internalize that phrase and think, "yes, maybe I can do this." Next, I considered the experiences that I had during my various fieldwork affiliations. Allow me an aside here to get on my soapbox and offer my opinion regarding fieldwork. It is imperative that you make the most of every minute and take advantage of the professionals around you. Through fieldwork, you are able to hone your clinical reasoning skills, receive constructive feedback, and begin to grow as a professional. Clinical reasoning is the foundation upon which the certification exam is built, so work with your supervisors and other staff to develop these skills. My feeling with school, fieldwork, and basically every aspect of life, is that you get out of it what you put in, so make the most of every moment. This will help you beyond measure to succeed, both in the exam room, and in practice. With that as my mindset, I used my fieldwork experiences to supplement the information within the various categories I had created.

The next step for me involved gathering as much information as I could about the test itself. Knowing the composition of the categories and weight that each section held guided me in determining which areas I needed to further supplement. I did this through the NBCOT Web site, along with a variety of different study guides. The value of the study guides, such as the previous edition of this text, was immeasurable in preparing for the exam. I understood that these study guides were not "real" tests, but were designed to help me think about questions. I immediately began taking the exams offered in the books. I only completed a portion of each exam at a time, so that I did not become overwhelmed with the information. That helped me to know in which areas I had a solid grasp, and in which areas I should focus more attention. Taking that first study exam was a brave and harrowing experience. Realizing how much or how little I recalled in specific areas was an eye opener, but it provided me with a plan of attack. I decided that I needed to further supplement my areas of weakness by gathering additional information from textbooks and professional Web sites. The piles were increasing, but so were my knowledge base and my confidence. Once I had gathered all of the information, I fell back on the skills that helped me throughout school: I planned. I purchased a large desk size calendar. On each day, I wrote the categories or material that I wanted to get through that day. I wrote the topics in pen, because I knew that pencil would be too easy to erase and put off until a later date. The structure is what made me successful. I mixed up the information that I really needed to focus on with the information that I already had a handle on so that if I fell behind one day, I could easily catch up the next. I then used a thick, black, permanent marker to cross out each area that I completed. There are few things that feel as good as the sense of accomplishment and confidence you feel as the black marks begin to predominate the calendar.

I completed one-half of a study exam each week. Most guides provide rationale for correct answers, together with outlining why the other options were incorrect. I completed the pencil and paper tests so that I could look back at them as part of my studying. Many of the books provide discs, which are helpful in providing a testing experience more similar to the actual exam. I am a concrete person, so being able to refer back to the paper exam was the most effective for me.

Another strategy I used was to go on-line and read postings and messages from other people who had taken the exam. One day when I was looking for information on the exam, I typed in NBCOT into the search engine. What I found was a network of people, much like myself, who were about to take the exam, or had recently received their results. This was very affirming because it let me know that I was not alone, and pass or fail, I would not be the first, or the last, to do either. I also found success stories, much like the one I am now able to write, with advice, opinions, and lists of useful resources. This was an extremely valuable tool that I had no idea existed. It was like a secret society of OT students. There was no secret handshake, but the camaraderie that developed between people that have shared the same pleasure, and pain, was invaluable. This is where I get on my soapbox again. As students, we live two lives—one with our home families, and one with our school families. Both of these are essential to your success. I will not expound upon the value of a good base of support at home. I think that that is well documented. However, I will tout the importance of your school family. Only an OT student knows what it is like to be an OT student. No one else has walked in those shoes, no matter what other professional degrees they may hold. Use that bond to work together to plan, study, or share materials, or to vent to someone who knows.

When my exam date was approximately 6 weeks away, I began taking the NBCOT practice exams on-line. There is a fee for these, however for me, it was money well spent. These exams are comprised of 100 questions, are timed, and are set up in a similar fashion to the actual exam, with the same percentage of questions in each domain as appear on the full exam. You receive the results right away, with an outline of your performance in each of the domains. The only negative aspect is that there is no breakdown of correct and incorrect responses, so you do not know which questions you answered correctly, nor do you receive a rationale for specific answers. This is the reason that it is important to use a variety of sources.

NBCOT permits a person to take three on-line practice exams, so I spread these out over the next few weeks. I saved the last one for the week before my scheduled exam, figuring it would give me a confidence boost if I did well, or outline the final area(s) that still needed attention if I did poorly. Luckily, it was the former rather than the latter, which put a small dent in the growing anxiety as the date approached. Ultimately, the score that I achieved on each of the three practice exams was almost identical to that which I scored on the actual exam.

When I scheduled my exam, I decided to schedule it for a Tuesday. That was a conscious decision. I figured that I would have the weekend to lock myself behind that previously closed door, within the room in which my presence amongst the piles of school "stuff" had become commonplace over the past several weeks. I thought I would then take Monday to relax and recuperate in preparation for the big day. Of course, this was wishful thinking. At that point, it is difficult to shut down because all you can think about is absorbing as much information as you can. In hindsight, I should have stuck with the original plan. What I had not learned up to that day would not have made as much a difference as a good night's sleep might have made. Knowing my personal study habits, however, I needed to take advantage of each minute to study in order to feel comfortable. Also, knowing that I am more of a morning person, I decided to schedule the exam first thing in the morning. It is important to have a good sense of yourself when making exam preparations in order to achieve the best outcome.

Some important things to consider when scheduling the exam are the location of the testing center, the time of day you want to take it, and the route you will take to get there. If you are unfamiliar with the area, take a trial run on the same day of the week and time that you have scheduled the exam so that you can get a sense of how much traffic there will be on that day and how much time it will take to get there. Then, add an extra 20 to 30 minutes just in case of an emergency. There is nothing worse than having something unforeseen happen, and then have to rush to get to the testing center. There is enough stress related to taking the exam under ideal circumstances.

Also, although your stomach may feel like it is auditioning for the Olympic tumbling team, try to eat something. The author of this study guide offered me some words of wisdom in that regard. Try to eat some carbohydrates (sorry Atkins' Diet fans). You are like an athlete running a 4-hour marathon, and you want to make sure that you have enough energy to reach the finish line. Also, try to get that rest that I mentioned. You want to give your brain, and body, time to oxygenate, and rejuvenate. Having a clear and focused mind is essential.

As you drive, listen to your favorite CD or radio station. This will give your mind a break. Some people prefer quiet during the ride, but I found that this made my mind wander into areas of uncertainty, and that is the last thing that I wanted in my head before the exam. In addition, when you arrive at the testing center, try not to take the closest parking space. Find a spot that will require a little walking. We all know the value of exercise in allowing the nervous system to calm and organize. As you walk, take some deep breaths and really draw the oxygen into your lungs. Your body and brain will thank you. Extra materials are not permitted into the testing area, but leave yourself a treat in the car. Chocolate works great for this! You will need something comforting once you are finished, and you should be rewarded for all of your hard work!

My testing center provided both earplugs and headphones for the exam. All provide one or the other, if not both. Use at least one of them. It will allow you to concentrate, and not be distracted by any sounds that are around you. Also, try not to consume too much liquid before the exam. You are permitted to go to the restroom, but your time continues to run. If you are typically a coffee drinker, make sure you have at least a small cup; otherwise you may end up with a caffeine withdrawal headache.

As you are taking the exam, go through and answer as many questions as you can. Mark the ones that you are not sure of or just want to go back and recheck. Be sure to read each question carefully. Sometimes the question asks for the MOST likely answer, and sometimes it asks for the LEAST likely. Take your time and read every word. Also, pay some attention to the clock, but do not become obsessed by the time. It is good to be aware of where you stand, but you cannot let it distract you. I found it helpful to plan to average about one minute per question. That left me approximately 40 minutes to go back and check the questions I marked. Some questions took much less than one minute, but some took more.

When you finish the exam, it is important to not start second-guessing yourself. Go back to the car and enjoy your special treat. Whether you have left yourself that chocolate, or something healthier, such as a new CD, savor every minute and try not to dwell on the questions. This is easier said than done, because the only questions that will be running through your mind are the ones that you are not sure you answered correctly. For me, the ones that I found easy were long forgotten, and all that I could think about were the ones that I found more difficult. This led me to convince myself that I had failed. I began making contingency plans for when I received the inevitable results. The only thing on my mind was what I would do WHEN, not IF I failed. I tried to put my mind on other things, but it invariably came back to the test. Although I questioned several of my responses, I avoided opening a single textbook or looking at any of my notes. To me, the uncertainty was better than the possibility of confirming that I had answered questions incorrectly.

Each day that passes while awaiting the test results are like an eternity. You find yourself completing busy work just to occupy your mind. It is a good idea to plan something fun for this time, such as a vacation or day trips. Any distraction is a blessing. For me, my friends and family tried to provide the moral support that I intrinsically lacked. I was showered with their confidence in me, but it really did little to help. How could they be so confident, when I was not? I write this not to cause any additional fear or reservation to that which you may already be experiencing, but to let you know that post-test anxiety is normal, and something that each of us that have been there has experienced. After you take the exam, I recommend rereading these pages. There is comfort in knowing that what you are feeling is typical, and that each of us has experienced the same emotions.

The day that the results arrived could not come too quickly for me, but even when it did, I was not quite ready. The culmination of all of the years of school and months of studying rested in my very shaky hands. There is nothing that prepares you for the roller coaster of emotions that you experience at that very moment. You engage in a sublime conversation with yourself deciding whether or not to open the letter. The minutes tick by, but you are not aware of their passage, transfixed only on the envelope until the need to know finally overtakes you.

The anxiety that made my hands tremble was quickly replaced by exuberance as I read the paper that began with "Congratulations…" There is little to compare to the feeling of elation at reading that single word. Being on the threshold of a career path that I love has made ever second of work worthwhile. It has been said that anything worth having is worth working for, and this is no exception. It is a tremendous task that is ahead of you as you begin this process, but remember that success is within your grasp and your future is an open door.

COUNTDOWN CALENDAR

A blank calendar is provided on page 11 to help you organize your last month before the exam. Use this calendar to chart your goals and study plans. Begin by entering the month and year you will take the exam. Enter the dates in each box and highlight your exam appointment. Remove the calendar from this book and post it in a prominent place. Once you have a dated calendar for your goals, you can begin to develop your study plans in Chapter Two.

SUMMARY

Beginning to study for the certification exam can be overwhelming. Information on where to start is provided in this chapter. The role of NBCOT, the history, and the process of the exam are reviewed to help you understand the exam. General study techniques and a countdown calendar are provided to guide you through your exam preparation. Information for creating a smooth exam day is also provided.

COUNTDOWN CALENDAR						
Sunday	Monday	Tuesday	Wednesday	Thursday	Friday	Saturday

SECTION II
Study Techniques

Chapter Two

Preparation and Studying to Meet the Challenge

Lori S. Gilmore, MS, CSE

GETTING STARTED

Congratulations! You have been successful in your coursework and are preparing to face the next challenge. Although your level of concern may be heightened, take a moment to inventory what you have accomplished. You have proven to yourself and your instructors that you are a capable learner, you have spent countless hours juggling coursework and other responsibilities, and you have gained new experiences to add to your repertoire. You are nearing the end of one phase of your formal education; no one can take away your accomplishment. Take a bow. With that feather in your hat, you are prepared to meet your next goal—passing the NBCOT exam.

The OTA exam may prove to be a unique studying experience for you. Pre-professionals from all over the country are taking the same exam as you. This may be the first time that you are expected to take an exam that is not related to one particular course. Although you have some hints of what to study, your preparation may need to be adjusted to be ready for a global test. You probably do not need a *how-to* study guide because you have already been successful. However, you may wish to look at your current study habits and determine whether you can be a more efficient learner. Perhaps there is a study technique that you have not thought of or a memory strategy that can benefit you. The purpose of this chapter is to help you select the study techniques that will be of most benefit to you as you prepare for the NBCOT exam.

You are in charge. No one will know if you are at the library studying or reading a magazine. You are responsible for your own study plan. Although studying can be a burden, its benefits outweigh the sacrifice. Not only does thoughtful preparation increase your knowledge base, but it also helps you to gain confidence, independence, and control. Although you may be missing out on other important activities, your situation is only temporary, and there will be a time when other goals will take priority. Effective studying will give you satisfaction, and you will know that no matter what the outcome, you have done your best and can hold your head high.

Remember, you are a unique individual. Do not waste time comparing yourself to others studying for the exam. Your experiences and personal situations are different from those of others. Accept your personal strengths and weaknesses, and develop a plan of attack based on your needs. Listen to others' good suggestions, but stick to the plan that will be of most benefit to *you*. Be honest in your own assessments and be willing to admit if something is not working. Evaluate your plan regularly to see if you are obtaining the results you intended. If not, modify your plan based on what you need.

Take the time now to make a plan. Even if it is a lousy one, you are heading in the right direction. You can always change it later, but at least move forward by making some decisions. The following pages will assist you in assessing your current learning preferences so that you may be able to develop an effective plan.

FINDING YOUR BEST LEARNING STYLE

Learning styles refer to the way people take in, store, and retrieve information. Some people learn and remember best by hearing, while others learn best by writing things out. You may have a preference for one style or modality; you may find that a combination of styles works best for you. Take the following inventory to help determine your strongest learning preference. Check the following characteristics that best apply to you.

LEARNING STYLE CHARACTERISTICS CHECKLIST

1. ___When I have a problem, I usually tell someone right away.
2. ___I keep a journal.
3. ___I often take notes, although I do not always refer to them.
4. ___I take good notes and then rewrite them at a later time.
5. ___I read in my free time.
6. ___I have the TV on even if I am not watching it.
7. ___I have good intentions of writing to people but usually call instead.
8. ___To help me concentrate, I often shut my eyes.
9. ___When studying or solving a problem, I pace back and forth.
10. ___I would rather hear a book on audiocassette than read it.
11. ___Forget the cassette, I would rather wait until it comes out on film.
12. ___I prefer reading the newspaper to watching the news on TV.
13. ___I prefer to study in a quiet setting.
14. ___To remember a spelling, I "see" the word in my mind.
15. ___I would prefer an oral exam to a written one.
16. ___I prefer a multiple-choice format on a test.
17. ___I would rather do a project than write a paper.
18. ___I would rather give an oral report than a written one.
19. ___I better remember what I read rather than what I hear.
20. ___I keep a personal organizer.
21. ___I reread my notes several times.
22. ___I would rather take notes from the text than attend a lecture on the material.
23. ___I often "talk" to myself.
24. ___I learn best when I study with a partner.
25. ___I can locate a passage that I have read by "seeing" it.
26. ___I find it hard to sit still when I study.
27. ___If I forget why I walked into the kitchen, I retrace my steps from the bedroom.
28. ___Once in bed for the night, I shut my eyes and plan the next day.
29. ___I cannot clean unless the music is on.
30. ___I would rather read directions than have someone tell me about them.
31. ___I can put something together as long as the directions are written.

SCORING THE CHECKLIST

Compare the answers from your checklist to the checklist below. Circle the letters that correspond to the items you marked.

1. S When I have a problem, I usually tell someone right away.
2. W I keep a journal.
3. M W I often take notes, although I do not always refer to them.
4. W I take good notes and then rewrite them at a later time.
5. R I read in my free time.
6. L I have the TV on even if I am not watching it.
7. S I have good intentions of writing to people but usually call instead.
8. V To help me concentrate, I often shut my eyes.
9. M When studying or solving a problem, I pace back and forth.
10. L I would rather hear a book on audiocassette than read it.

11.	V	Forget the cassette, I would rather wait until it comes out on film.
12.	R	I prefer reading the newspaper to watching the news on TV.
13.	L	I prefer to study in a quiet setting.
14.	V	To remember a spelling, I "see" the word in my mind.
15.	S	I would prefer an oral exam to a written one.
16.	V	I prefer a multiple choice format on a test.
17.	M	I would rather do a project than write a paper.
18.	S	I would rather give an oral report than a written one.
19.	R	I better remember what I read rather than what I hear.
20.	W	I keep a personal organizer.
21.	R	I reread my notes several times.
22.	W	I would rather take notes from the text than attend a lecture on the material.
23.	S L	I often "talk" to myself.
24.	S L	I learn best when I study with a partner.
25.	V	I can locate a passage that I have read by "seeing" it.
26.	M	I find it hard to sit still when I study.
27.	M	If I forget why I walked into the kitchen, I retrace my steps from the bedroom.
28.	V	Once in bed for the night, I shut my eyes and plan the next day.
29.	L	I cannot clean unless the music is on.
30.	R	I would rather read directions than have someone tell me about them.
31.	R	I can put something together as long as the directions are written.

Tally the number of S, W, M, R, L, and V responses, and record the total in the following table.

LEARNING STYLE CHARACTERISTICS CHECKLIST

S	W	M	R	L	V

If you have three or more responses of one letter, you most likely have a strong preference for that learning style. Most people have at least one strength, but you may have more than one strong area.

RESULTS

Speaking (S): Three or more checks in this area indicate a preference for learning information by saying it. You may wish to read your notes and text aloud or at least the chapter headings. It may be beneficial for you to have a study partner or to speak into a tape recorder and play your tape back. You may ask someone to listen to you as you explain a principle. After reviewing information, play the part of a teacher by asking questions aloud. Repeat concepts aloud and ask questions of others.

Writing (W): Take notes from readings. Rewrite your notes on paper or index cards. Make tests for yourself and then take them. Write notes in the margins of your texts and notebooks.

Manipulative (M): Often thought of as the kinesthetic modality, learning occurs best by "doing." If you have this type of preference, make a model, map, or diagram of information you need to learn. Write information on a black/white board. Carry index cards with the information you are trying to learn with you, and pull out the cards while you are walking, exercising, or cooking dinner. "Draw" answers in the air as you try to memorize information. Move your lips while you are reading or thinking.

Reading (R): Read and reread information if this is your preferred learning style. Ask others for their notes so you can read them and fill in any information you have missed. Highlight text passages to easily locate information. Read chapter titles, headings, and summaries.

Listening (L): You would benefit from having a study group or at least a partner. To the extent possible, have others read to you. Tape lectures and review sessions when possible. Make review tapes for yourself and then listen to them. Read and repeat information aloud after you have read or heard it. Call classmates and have them read their notes to you or quiz you over the phone.

Visualizing (V): If this is your learning strength, you learn best by picturing information in your head. You are apt to "see" a page of information. It is to your benefit to study, then shut your eyes and recall the information. Take note of the way the information is written and the shape, color, size of the paper, etc. to help you recall the information later. You can also picture yourself taking the exam, walking in, and calmly sitting down. This will help to steady your nerves.

Often, it is beneficial for you to study in more than one way. Remember, your learning profile is unique, and just because your friend studies best when listening to music does not mean that the same will apply to you. Take a moment to inventory your strengths, and develop a plan based on the way you learn best.

GETTING ORGANIZED TO STUDY

How much time do you have to study, or how much time are you willing to give based on your work schedule, information retained from classes, anxiety level, and other commitments? Fill out the following time log to visually see how you have been spending your time. If possible, do this for several days, including a weekend day.

TIME LOG			
Day			
6:00-7:00 a.m.			
7:00-8:00			
8:00-9:00			
9:00-10:00			
10:00-11:00			
11:00-12:00 noon			
12:00-1:00 p.m.			
1:00-2:00			
2:00-3:00			
3:00-4:00			
4:00-5:00			
5:00-6:00			
6:00-7:00			
7:00-8:00			
8:00-9:00			
9:00-10:00			
10:00-11:00			

Based on how your time is usually spent, what available time do you have for studying? Will you be better off studying for a block of time in the afternoon or for several chunks throughout the day? Perhaps your schedule is such that you can only realistically study on weekends. How much time can you commit to studying during your free time? Based on the amount of time you have, make a plan (you can always modify it later) of when you are going to study.

STUDY TIME COMMITMENTS

Next, make a list of the supplies you need for studying. This may sound silly, but it is a necessary physical and mental process that will help prepare you for the task itself. Besides, it's more pleasant to study if you have colored index cards and a candy supply.

STUDY SUPPLIES	
Suggested Study Supplies	*Your List of Study Supplies*
Reference books (*DSM IV*, guides, dictionary, etc.)	
Different colored index cards	
Index cards on a wire	
Notetabs	
Different colored highlighters	
Timer/clock	
Goal sheet: long- and short-term	
Writing instruments	
Tissues	
Water or juice	

STUDY SUPPLIES (CONTINUED)	
Suggested Study Supplies	*Your List of Study Supplies*
Tape recorder	
Lined/unlined paper	
Snacks or treats (granola bars, mints, crackers, etc.)	
Tools of the trade (goniometer, etc.)	
Class notes, prior exams if available	
Rabbit's foot or other good luck charms	

Stock your study area with the supplies you determined were needed. If you travel to the library or study in several different places, prepare a bag with your supplies so you will always have them at hand. Note: if you have run out of mints more than three times, you need to reevaluate your priorities.

Now that you have determined when you will study and your needed supplies, you are ready to make a plan of attack. Begin by developing a goal sheet for yourself. Examine the sample below as a guideline for your goal sheet.

SAMPLE GOAL SHEET			
Outcome goal: To pass the NBCOT exam and become an OTA.			
Current Date	*Objectives*	*Target Completion Date*	*Revision of Goals or Progress Notes*
11/30	Complete 30 questions from review manual	11/30	Done. Got 23 correct.
12/1	Photocopy Amy's notes on TBI; give her a copy of my SCI notes	12/2	
12/4	Read chapter summaries in text books	12/4	Took longer than expected. Finish 12/5.
12/6	Make flashcards/vocabulary cards	12/6	Ran out of cards. Go shopping by 12/8.
12/9	Tape record content outline from text	12/11	Done. Victorious. Yahoo for me!
12/10	Finish vocabulary cards	12/10	Done. Pat self on the back.
12/12	Highlight vocabulary in text	12/15	Finished 12/13. See a movie.
12/15	Reorganize notebook	12/16	No interest. Try again.
12/16	Form a study group	12/18	No problem.
12/17	Reorganize notebook	12/18	Watched *Frosty the Snowman* instead.
12/19	Reorganize notebook	12/19	Maybe tomorrow.

Now complete your goal sheet.

GOAL SHEET

Outcome goal:

Current Date	Objectives	Target Completion Date	Revision of Goals or Progress Notes

Review and revise your plan of attack often. If nothing else, remove the sheet from the book and post it where it will remind you that you do have a goal in mind. Be flexible. Your great-aunt may stop over (and you know what that means), or you may find yourself completing goals ahead of schedule.

Make goals reasonable. It is unrealistic to expect yourself to complete 300 review questions in an hour, yet completing five vocabulary flashcards per week is no great accomplishment. Base your goals on the amount of overall time you have (and are willing) to study. Chapter One has a countdown calendar to help you set your goals.

SPECIFIC STUDY AND TEST SKILLS

It is recommended that you look at specific study and test skills that can improve your chances of identifying the correct answer on the NBCOT exam. Since the examination will be computerized beginning in September 2001, it may be helpful to think about the following skills with the idea that you will be reading from a computer screen.

Reading comprehension: Points on the exam are not awarded for how long you study, your effort, or the amount of pages you read. Generally, grades are earned by knowing the correct information. It is quite important that you have good comprehension of the material you are reading. The following are suggestions to aid in understanding your reading material: preview the chapter you are about to read by scanning the title, headings, introduction, summary, and, on occasion, the topic sentence in each paragraph. This can be helpful in reviewing a chapter or passage you have already read. Take regular breaks to mentally review what you have read. Turn topic sentences into questions. Answer these in your head or jot them down for later review. Read the material carefully, checking your understanding as you go along.

Note taking: Taking notes on materials that you are studying can be beneficial. Remember, even if you never review the notes you take, the process of jotting them down can be helpful. Outlining with a highlighter may help zero in on the main idea. If this method works well for you, use a different colored marker to highlight the details or supporting ideas. Reread your highlighted passages. Class notes as well as textbooks can be highlighted. Use margin notes to organize what you have read. Pay attention to key words, or write questions in the margin for later review. Margin notes will help avoid wasted time searching for an answer because the explanation will be right near the notes.

Another way to take notes on important material is to jot down information in a separate notebook. Again, this is particularly helpful for those who learn best kinesthetically. Note taking should always be done by using phrases rather than complete sentences. Make an informal outline by writing down the main idea from a passage and several supporting details under the idea. Always jot down the page number or source of information so you can refer back to it if needed.

If you have found that you remember information best by picturing the words on a page or by writing, then you might consider mapping as a note-taking strategy. Draw a circle in the middle of your page and write the main idea in it. Write the major points regarding your main topic on connecting lines. This might include information such as causes and effects or symptoms and treatments. Add lines to your major points to connect minor details. See Figure 2-1 as an example.

Lastly, notes can be written on index cards. Put one key concept and supporting details on each notecard. Reference your card so you know where to find additional information should you have a question. Write down pertinent vocabulary to the concept. If there is a definition associated with your concept, write that on the back of your card so you can test yourself. One advantage to using notecards is the opportunity to put a few in your pocket to review while you are waiting in the car, or to stick on your mirror while you blow dry your hair, or to view on the refrigerator as you contemplate a snack.

Memory strategies: Comprehending the material you hear and read is one thing, but memorizing it is another. Fortunately, most of what is asked of us deals more with integrating and applying information rather than memorizing long lists of terms. However, there are occasions when you will be responsible for producing an exact definition, listing the components of a subject, or remembering several general concepts. Unfortunately, most of us have more difficulty memorizing information than we did when we were younger. Not to worry. If you can recite the alphabet, then you should be able to remember just about anything. Consider all the similar sounding letters in the alphabet (B, C, D, E, G, P, T, V, Z) yet, even with confusing sounds, we have mastered the ABCs. Most likely, you were able to learn the alphabet because of repetition, repetition, and repetition. Chances are you know a little tune whereby you can sing the ABCs on demand. The same strategies, plus some others, that worked when you were 5 years old can work for you now.

We are constantly taking in information, but the degree to which we remember or retrieve the information depends on several factors. Exposure or repetition is definitely a factor that affects our ability to remember an item. For instance, fill in the following:

"Here's George Jetson, Jane, his _____."

"That's the way we became the _____ Bunch."

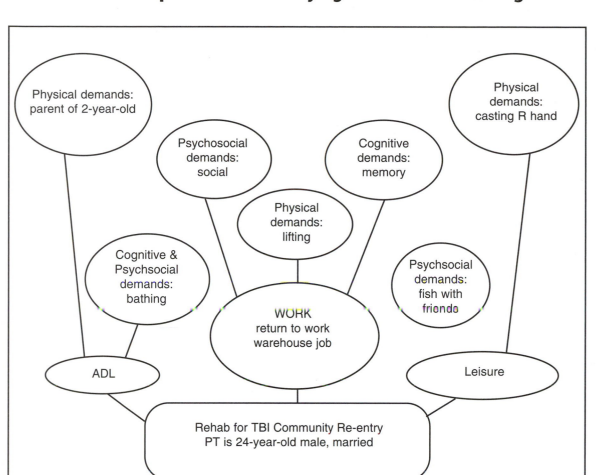

Figure 2-1. Occupational therapy mapping example (reprinted with permission from Sladyk, K., McGeary, S., Sladyk, LG., & Tufano, R. (2001). *OT exam review manual* (3rd ed.). Thorofare, NJ: SLACK Incorporated).

"It takes one to _____ one."

"I've been _____ on the railroad."

You have heard these phrases over and over until you automatically know the answers. Over-learning is an effective way to move information from your short-term memory to your long-term knowledge. Read and re-read the information you are trying to memorize. Once you feel you have learned the material, review it regularly to refresh your memory. Each time you review the material, it will take less and less time until you can anticipate words and phrases before you even read them. As you review material, recite it so you can see and hear the information. Writing and rewriting (more than once) will help you to retain information. Try to link new information with prior knowledge.

Use rhymes, acronyms, acrostics, and substitutions in familiar sayings or tunes. For instance, if you are trying to memorize the joints in the hands (MCP, PIP, DIP), you might memorize **My Cousin Paul Put Ice Pieces Down Ida's Pants**. Rearrange items in your list (unless they have to be remembered in a specific order) to make it easier to work with.

Break down long lists of vocabulary into smaller, manageable chunks. For instance, if you have 120 terms that you need to learn or review, divide the list into six groups of 20 terms. Put 100 terms out of reach and concentrate only on 20 terms at a time. Begin by reviewing the first term. Next study the second term. Next study the first term again, and review the second term. Now you can add the third term. Before looking at the fourth term, review the first three terms. Get it? After awhile, you will become quite proficient at identifying the first few terms. Your speed will increase as you anticipate the answers. Your confidence will build, and you will remember far more than you would have if you went through all 20 (or 120) terms at once.

Test-taking strategies: Know the format of the test. It is easier to prepare when you know what the expectations are. For instance, on an essay test you will have to retrieve information and do so in an orderly way. You will need to know pertinent vocabulary and how to use it appropriately. However, the reason you're reading this book is because of a specific multiple-choice test in the near future. A multiple-choice format is advantageous in that you need only to recognize the correct answer rather than generate it yourself. Still, there are techniques that will enhance your chances of choosing the correct answer. The following are some tactics that will:

A. Help you to buy a new car

B. Help you lose 10 pounds

C. Better clean your house

D. Help you succeed on the big test

The correct answer is D, though with your increased confidence, you may increase your likelihood of meeting the other goals. The following test-taking strategies will help you succeed on the exam:

- Plan your time: Divide your time by the number of questions. Leave several minutes leeway.

- Read the entire question: Anticipate the answer but do not be impulsive. Read each answer thoroughly before choosing.

- Respond to each question: If you leave it blank, it is definitely wrong. If you have absolutely no clue, then make the best guess possible.

- If you are unsure of the answer: Narrow it down by eliminating the responses you know are incorrect. Sometimes you can get clues from reading other questions.

- Pay particular attention to qualifying words: Words such as except, most, best, least, and not.

- Do not over-interpret the questions: Read them at face value.

- If you do not know the right answer: Make the best response possible and put a check by the question. If you have the time, return to the question to recheck.

- Do not waste time on the questions you do not know.

- If you must skip a question: you can flag an unanswered question and return to it later. Again, you are better off answering all the questions and flagging the ones you want to check later.

- Continually check to make sure you have keyed in the answers correctly: Make sure the number of your question corresponds to the number on your answer sheet.

- After September 2001, all applicants will be taking a computerized test unless requesting special accommodations for pencil and paper. If you do use paper and pencil, color in the bubbles carefully: Do not overdo it. Erase wrong answers completely.

- Trust your instincts: Do not second guess yourself. Be cautious about changing answers.

- Check the time: Check the clock or your watch occasionally to make sure you are on target.

- Remind yourself how great you are.

READY TO STUDY

With supplies at hand, snacks in stock, and goal sheet pinned to your chest, you are ready to get down and dirty. Before you sit down, you need to decide on a place for your intellectual experience (a.k.a study environment). Consider the amount of noise, light, temperature, and physical comfort of your study area. In addition, will there be visual interference that will cause you to look up every few moments? Is your studying most effective morning, noon, or night? Make these decisions now to maximize your effectiveness.

Refer to your goal list to set expectations for each particular study session. Be aware that the first few minutes of your session are considered warm-up time, which you will spend "shifting gears" and getting in the right mindset. Monitor your progress to check for fatigue and mind wandering. Evaluate your session afterward to see if you were effective or if you need to change something for next time. Refer to the following study session evaluation checklist:

- Did I have specific goals in mind as I sat to study?

- Were my expectations realistic?

- Did I accomplish what I set out to do?

- Was the time I set aside sufficient?

- Did I implement specific study techniques based on my preferred learning style?

- Was I distracted or tired?

TROUBLE SHOOTING

If your efforts are sincere but you are not getting the results you desire, refer to the following problem-solving solutions.

TROUBLE-SHOOTING SOLUTIONS	
If	Try
You are sleepy	Physical activity, a break, a real nap, fresh air, a study partner, speaking aloud.
Your mind wanders	A new location; earplugs; set smaller, more obtainable goals; use manipulatives.
You are bored	Vary your routine; give yourself rewards; try 15 minutes on, 15 minutes off; switch from reading to writing to speaking.
You have too many interruptions	Take the phone off the hook/put the answering machine on, put up a sign that says "Great mind at work—please do not interrupt."
You are worried, overwhelmed	Break tasks down to even smaller chunks, see relaxation strategies.
You are forgetting previously learned material	Use clues to get information flowing, review less material more frequently, do not move to new concepts until old concepts are mastered, try learning through a different modality.
You are behind on your goals	Reevaluate your time, double up on goals, refer to Chapter One for the countdown calendar.

RELAXATION TECHNIQUES AND COPING SKILLS

As an occupational therapy assistant student you have learned that relaxation techniques are effective for helping your patients cope. Studying for the exam is a good time to use relaxation exercises yourself. The following exercises may be effective both before and during the exam.

Self talk: Ask yourself what is the worst thing that will happen if...

—you do not study tonight?

—you do not pass the test?

Tell yourself that you can do this. You have done other hard things and can do this too. You are great!

Review successes: Remind yourself of previous successes. You have made it this far; you have passed all your courses. You have passed other examinations. You have completed a successful affiliation.

Take inventory: Do you know more than you did last year? Do you know more than you did last month? Have you studied/reviewed material recently?

Develop support systems: Let people know of your goals. Phone others to discuss your concerns (avoid calling Patty Perfect). Be with people who will validate your self-worth.

Visualization: Picture yourself walking into the exam with confidence. Visualize yourself getting the results in the mail and scoring in the top 20%.

Daydream: Think about tanning on the beach or skiing down a slope. Take a vacation in your mind.

Have a pity party: Get the whining over with. Invite others to come over and see who can complain the most. After everyone is done complaining, consider a short study group.

Physical activity: Walking can clear your head and relax your muscles. Elevate your feet by lying on the floor and placing your feet on a chair for 10 minutes.

Deep breathing: Try deep cleansing breaths. Shut your eyes and slowly inhale through your nose. Hold the breath for 3 to 5 seconds and then exhale through your mouth. Repeat every time you feel stressed. If you are familiar with meditation techniques, try them after a few deep cleansing breaths.

SUMMARY

There is satisfaction in knowing that you have done your best. The ideas presented in this chapter are suggestions in how to help you reach your goal of preparing, studying, and ultimately passing your examination. Preparing to study according to your strengths and weaknesses is an important part of studying effectively. Information regarding learning styles, organization, and specific study strategies is included in this chapter. It is important to develop the strategies that will be of most benefit to you. A study plan will ultimately help you save time and learn efficiently and effectively.

Chapter Three

Content Study Outlines

Occupational therapy "content" is all the things you learned in OTA school. A person studying for the NBCOT exam might want to develop a content study outline to structure the studying process.

There are many ways to review the material that is on the NBCOT exam. NBCOT provides a matrix on exam material already mentioned in Chapter One of this book and available online at www.nbcot.org. The NBCOT outline includes human development, treatment implementation, etc., but many students find the outline vague. A second way to review for the exam is to make up a study outline using your class syllabi and notes. A third way is to use the table of contents in major OTA textbooks. Although it is not recommended that you try to reread your textbooks, you will find the table of contents helpful in organizing your studying. A fourth way to organize your study outline is to use resource books such as Sladyk's *OT Study Cards in a Box* or Reed's *Quick Reference to Occupational Therapy*. Both of these books are listed in Appendix A. Lastly, a study outline is provided here for your convenience. This content study outline is adapted from *Ryan's Occupational Therapy Assistant, Third Edition*. It provides a holistic and across the age span look at OTA practice.

FOUNDATIONS OF OCCUPATIONAL THERAPY

I. History of Occupation
   A. Key concepts: moral treatment, purposeful activity

II. Philosophy and Core Values
   A. Key concepts: occupation, meaningful activities, quality of life

III. Normal Human Development
   A. Key concepts: Piaget, Erickson, Maslow, Freud
   B. OTA concerns: all developmental milestones in physical, emotional, and social development from birth to old age

IV. Anatomy
   A. Key concepts: structure and function of body systems, muscle function, types of joints, and connective tissues
   B. OTA concerns: inflammation, edema, pain

V. *Practice Framework*
   A. Key concept: language of occupational therapy
   B. OTA concerns: all occupational performance areas, skills, and contexts

VI. Activity Analysis
   A. Key concept: tool of occupational therapy
   B. OTA concerns: analysis of each task, adaptation of tasks, gradation of tasks, therapeutic potential

VII. Theories and Frames of Reference
   A. Key concept: provide structure to treatment
   B. OTA concerns: basic knowledge of the role of theory in treatment. General: model of human occupation, person-environment-occupation, occupational performance, occupational science, Canadian Model of Occupational Performance. Physical function: biomechanical, neurodevelopmental, rehabilitation, proprioceptive neuromuscular facilitation. Psychosocial function: role acquisition, behavioral, cognitive, cognitive-behavioral, object relations, humanistic. Pediatrics: sensory integration, developmental, motor learning, spatiotemporal adaptation. Cognitive: cognitive perceptual, cognitive disabilities

VIII. Therapeutic Intervention Process
   A. Key concepts: referral, screening, evaluation, assessment, treatment planning, treatment implementation, re-evaluation, program discontinuation

IX. Teaching and Learning in OT
   A. Key concepts: good communication, begin treatment where client is, acknowledge culture, active learning, control consequences, provide practice by trial and error, repetition, practice in different settings, move from simple to complex, encourage problem solving, acknowledge stress of learning

OCCUPATIONS AND DISABILITIES

I. Attention Deficit Hyperactivity Disorder (ADHD)
   A. Key concepts: inattention, high level of activity, disorganization, social skills, medications, diet changes
   B. OTA concerns: eligible under Individuals with Disabilities Education Act (IDEA) or 504, environmental adaptations especially seating, cognitive and social observations, organizing tasks, checklists, behavior management, possible home visit, as adults some symptoms may persist

II. Acquired Immunodeficiency Syndrome (AIDS) and Other Infectious Diseases
   A. Key concepts: immune disorder, opportunistic infections, weight loss, medications, universal precautions, hospice care
   B. OTA concerns: muscle tone and strength, fine and gross motor movement, cognitive skills, perceptual skills, coping and adjustment, quality of life issues, support system, community resources, environmental adaptations, energy conservation, sexual adjustment, activities of daily living (ADLs), work, leisure

III. Amputation
   A. Key concepts: diabetes, trauma, peripheral vascular disease, phantom pain, wound care
   B. OTA concerns: self-image, pre-prosthetic training, wound healing, skin and stump care, use versus cosmetic issues, scar massage, putting on and removing prosthetic, energy conservation and strengthening, environmental adaptations, community mobility, sexual adjustment, ADLs, work, leisure

IV. Anxiety
   A. Key concepts: stress reaction, agoraphobia, obsession, compulsion, panic, post-traumatic stress
   B. OTA concerns: assess suicidal thoughts, relaxation, cognitive-behavioral techniques such as desensitization, stress management, coping skills

V. Arthritis
   A. Key concepts: juvenile rheumatoid, rheumatoid, osteoarthritis, systemic versus not, inflammation versus not, exacerbation, remission, joint deformity, splinting, contractions, nonsteroidal anti-inflammatory drugs (NSAIDs)
   B. OTA concerns: joint protection, body mechanics, work simplification, adaptive equipment, energy conservation, rest versus exercise, environmental adaptations, community mobility, sexual adjustment, ADLs, work, leisure

VI. Bipolar Disorder
   A. Key concepts: manic and depressive extreme swings, often risky behaviors in manic stage with spending, dating, substances, or criminal activity, lithium most common medication
   B. OTA concerns: assess suicidal thoughts, develop insight and judgment, coping skills, self-control in social situations, ADLs, work and leisure affected

VII. Blindness
   A. Key concepts: blindness at birth (see low vision for older adults) may be from exposure to oxygen in premature infants, genetics, or pre-birth conditions, cataracts, retinopathy, myopia, strabismus, amblyopia, IDEA
   B. OTA concerns: physical, emotional, and social development including reflex maturation, sensory integration, stimulate remaining vision, balance, family-centered treatment, play, feeding, academic preparation and skills, compensatory strategies, work simplification and/or adaptive strategies in ADLs, work, leisure

VIII. Burns
   A. Key concepts: rule of nines, body surface, first degree—superficial, second degree—partial, third degree—full, fourth degree—electrical, debridement, grafts, respiratory and cardiac issues, shock, hypertrophic bone ossification
   B. OTA concerns: aseptic techniques, infection control, positioning, range of motion (ROM), scarring, position of comfort may cause deformity, contractures, splints, self-image, pain management, developmental issues if child, environmental adaptations, community mobility, sexual adjustment, ADLs, work, leisure

IX. Cancer
   A. Key concepts: computed tomography (CT) scans, magnetic resonance imaging (MRI), positron emission tomography (PET) scans improve diagnosis, prognosis varies by type and stage, metastasis, surgery, radiation, chemotherapy, nutrition, hospice
   B. OTA concerns: restorative, supportive, or palliative treatment; fatigue; energy conservation; ostomy care; pain management; family education; home and work site modifications; community support services; psychosocial issues

X. Cardiac Disease
   A. Key concepts: class I to IV for diagnosis related to impact on function (I is no impact, IV is impaired functioning), lifestyle history, shortness of breath, angina, metabolic equivalent (MET) levels, blood pressure, arrhythmia, dyspnea, chronic obstructive pulmonary disease (COPD)
   B. OTA concerns: lifestyle redesign, avocation, graded exercise, nutrition, stress management, work simplification, safety, sexual concerns

XI. Cerebral Palsy (CP)
   A. Key concepts: medical-based services versus educational-based services, spastic (most common), ataxia, athetoid, hypotonic, spasticity
   B. OTA concerns: neurodevelopmental treatment, reflex integration, family-centered treatment, learning disabilities, nystagmus, feeding issues, positioning, equilibrium, coordination, social skill development, sensory issues, may have mental retardation, vision problems

XII. Child/Elder Abuse
   A. Key concepts: impulse control of caregiver from personal, crisis, support, or difficult care factors; families usually have disorganized life; abuse may be physical, emotional, sexual, and/or financial
   B. OTA concerns: highly individualized, general developmental, physical and psychosocial assessment of needs, relaxation, coping skills, family focused, safety, advocacy, ADLs, work, leisure

XIII. Cerebrovascular Accident (CVA)
   A. Key concepts: dysarthria, expressive or receptive aphasia, apraxia, hemiparesis, flaccid, spastic tone, shoulder subluxation, visual issues including hemianopsia, subacute rehabilitation

B. OTA concerns: safety, muscle tone, and strength, ROM, sensory loss, synergy, positioning, neuro-developmental treatment (NDT), skin integrity, joint protection, safety, adaptive equipment, one-handed techniques, communication, family education, energy conservation, work simplification, wheelchair mobility, transfers, self-ROM, environmental adaptations, self-image, community mobility, sexual adjustment, driving, ADLs, work, leisure

XIV. Dementia
   A. Key concepts: brain dysfunction, caregiver roles, agnosia, aphasia, apraxia, memory, Alzheimer's disease, sundown syndrome
   B. OTA concerns: family education, consistent schedule, orientation when possible, validation when not, do not expect new learning, safety, strong lighting, quiet environment, play era music, use long-term memory in conversation, adapt environment, utilize pets, encourage exercise and socialization, help caregivers adjust, community resources

XV. Depression
   A. Key concepts: most common psychiatric disorder, family pattern possible, medication and side effects
   B. OTA concerns: assess suicidal thoughts, suicidal potential may increase as the person feels better, stress management, coping skills, relaxation, routine schedule, goal setting

XVI. Diabetes
   A. Key concepts: Sugar level, long-term effects on other organ systems.
   B. OTA concerns: lifestyle redesign, coping skills, stress management, relaxation, social skills training, developing new friendships and supports, leisure management, work

XVII. Drug/Alcohol Abuse
   A. Key concepts: lifestyle issues, 12-step programs, abstinence, detoxification, polysubstance abuse, recovery, sobriety
   B. OTA concerns: lifestyle redesign, coping skills, stress management, relaxation, social skills training, developing new friendships and supports, leisure management, work

XVIII. Eating Disorders
   A. Key concepts: anorexia nervosa, bulimia nervosa, medical issues including cardiac, possible family dysfunction, nutrition, dental and skin changes
   B. OTA concerns: assess suicidal thoughts, self-control, self-esteem, self-worth, perfectionism, social skills, and leisure

XIX. Hand/Arm Injuries
   A. Key concepts: carpal tunnel syndrome, fractures, cumulative trauma, peripheral nerve injuries, tendonitis, bursitis, scleroderma, tendon injuries, reflex sympathetic dystrophy
   B. OTA concerns: ROM, goniometry, volumetry for edema measurement, muscle strength and endurance, splinting, pain management, edema management, scar massage, coordination, dexterity, fine motor movement, work station evaluation and redesign, sensory retraining, graded exercise, adaptive equipment, body mechanics

XX. Head Injuries
   A. Key concepts: Rancho Los Amigos (RLA) levels I to VIII, coup and countercoup, frontal and temporal lobes, amnesia, coma, seizures, cranial nerves, other medical conditions
   B. OTA concerns: cognitive and sensory loss, visual perceptual changes, low vision, aphasia, splinting, behavioral changes, family education, motoric loss, balance, positioning, skin integrity, coordination, dysphagia, safety, ADLs, work, leisure, alcohol post injury, adaptive equipment, environmental adaptations, driving

XXI. Learning Disabilities
   A. Key concepts: inability to get, retain, or use skills due to poor memory, attention, or thinking; dyslexia; neurological impairments
   B. OTA concerns: reflex and motor development, fine and gross motor, motor planning, bilateral integration, visual-motor, postural control, perceptual skills, attention, self-control, academic development, sensory processing, problem solving, social skills

XXII. Low Vision and Hearing Loss
   A. Key concepts: legal blindness, low vision, visual impairments, vision rehabilitation, cataracts, diabetic retinopathy, glaucoma, macular degeneration, scotoma
   B. OTA concerns: spot reading, visual fields, center vision, environmental adaptations, adaptive equipment, safety, glare-free lighting, community resources, hearing aid refusal

XXIII. Mental Retardation
   A. Key issues: MR in adults over 18 (see pervasive development disorder [PDD] for children) have continued medical issues, dementia more common with some diagnoses
   B. OTA concerns: fine and gross motor, attention, developmental level, independence, splinter skills, interpersonal skills, adaptation of work site or sheltered work experience, coaching, community living skills including mobility, advocacy

XXIV. Multiple Sclerosis
   A. Key concepts: central nervous system (CNS) disorder, exacerbation, remission, mobility concerns
   B. OTA concerns: muscle weakness, incoordination, tremors, sensory issues, pain, visual problems, mood swings, cognitive involvement, home and work adaptations, safety, adaptive equipment, driving, ADLs, bladder problems may require self catheterization

XXV. Muscular Dystrophy
   A. Key concepts: progressive muscle weakness, pulmonary issues, Gowers' sign, lordosis, scoliosis, fat replaces muscle tissue, atrophy, cardiac issues
   B. OTA concerns: splinting and positioning to prevent contractures, gait problems or wheelchair mobility, family education, muscle imbalance, adaptive equipment, play development, home modifications, academic issues with possible cognitive problems

XXVI. Orthopedic Conditions
   A. Key concepts: hip fracture or replacement (arthroplasty or arthrodesis), knee fracture or replacement (see hand injuries for upper extremities [UE]), cognitive issues often temporarily common after hip surgery
   B. OTA concerns: muscle strength and endurance, ROM, hip precautions, dressing, toileting, bathing, mobility, safety, fear of falls, reacher bars installed in wall studs, adaptive equipment for hips but often not for knees, home modification

XXVII. Parkinson's Disease
   A. Key concepts: akinesia, bradykinesia, dopamine, dysarthria, festination, substantia nigra, tremors, rigidity, and stiffness of limbs and trunk
   B. OTA concerns: micrographia, postural instability, progressive resistive exercise, proprioceptive neuromuscular facilitation, safety, mobility, prevent deformities, communication, psychosocial adjustment, community support, ADLs, work, leisure

XXVIII. Personality Disorders
   A. Key concepts: inaccurate perception of self and others, often life-long
   B. OTA concerns: assess suicidal thoughts, values and goals development, relationship skills, suspicious types do best with individual treatment while others do best in groups, transference and counter-transference, work, leisure, social skills

XXIX. Pervasive Developmental Disorder
   A. Key concepts: infection, intoxication, trauma, nutrition or genetic causes, Rett syndrome, autism, Asperger's syndrome, along with mental retardation from a variety of causes
   B. OTA concerns: reflex and motor development, reflex integration, muscle tone, hand function, bilateral integration, feeding, motor planning, sensory issues, social roles, learning disabilities, play development, cognitive and academic issues, issues that continue through adulthood

XXX. Schizophrenia
   A. Key concepts: thought disorder, delusions, hallucinations, positive and negative symptoms, tardive dyskinesia, extrapyramidal symptoms, high smoking rate
   B. OTA concerns: assess suicidal thoughts, do not challenge or correct psychotic thinking, sensorimotor and cognitive treatment, behavioral techniques, ADLs, work, leisure

XXXI. Sensory Integration (SI) Dysfunction
   A. Key concepts: adaptive response, sensory defensiveness, overseas adoptions
   B. OTA concerns: auditory, tactile, olfactory, or visual defensiveness, dyspraxia, gravitational insecurity, ideation, impaired auditory processing, motor planning, praxis, proprioception, reflex integration, feeding, family-centered practice, academic issues, parent-child relationship, muscle strength, coordination, balance, vestibular stimulation

XXXII. Spina Bifida
   A. Key concepts: vertebral column does not close, hydrocephalus
   B. OTA concerns: muscle strength, tone, reflex maturation, movement, coordination, hand function, eye tracking, endurance, work tolerance, motor planning, sensory issues, perceptual skills, toileting

XXXIII. Spinal Cord Injuries
   A. Key concepts: spinal cord levels, autonomic dysreflexia, decubitus ulcers, heterotopic ossification, orthostatic hypotension, tetraplegia, paraplegia, respiratory impairment, decreased temperature regulation
   B. OTA concerns: tenodesis, self-catheterization, safety and precautions, ROM, skin integrity, self-ROM, sensory losses, splinting, wheelchair positioning, adaptive equipment, environmental modifications, community support, family education, sexual adjustment, driving, ADLs, work, leisure

Treatment Techniques, Procedures, and Concepts

I. Group Dynamics and Therapeutic Use of Self
   A. Key concepts: therapeutic relationship, group dynamics, group process, here and now focus, norms, roles, tasks, verbal and nonverbal communication
   B. OTA concerns: Fidler's task group, Mosey's developmental group, Kaplan's directive group, Ross' integrative group, Allen's cognitive levels, leadership styles, group membership, seven-stage activity group

II. Arts and Crafts
   A. OTA concerns: role of crafts, cooking, computers, etc., in meaningful activity

III. Assistive Technology
   A. Key concepts: equipment design process, safety, adaptive equipment, trial use, client acceptance, ease of use
   B. OTA concerns: only what the client needs and accepts

IV. Splinting
   A. Key concepts: biomechanical, fabrication techniques, client education, force, arches, function, static versus dynamic
   B. OTA concerns: typical goal is to maintain normal arches and neutral positions, neck conformer prevents contractures, axillary or airplane maintains abduction, elbow conformer maintains extension, cock-up maintains wrist flexion, resting hand maintains neutral, abductor wedge supports hip abduction, knee conformer maintains extension, foot drop maintains ankle in neutral

V. Wellness and Health Promotion
   A. Key concepts: health, wellness, Americans with Disabilities Act (ADA), ergonomics
   B. OTA concerns: lifestyle redesigned, health promotion, spirituality and hope, community wellness, community redesign, assistive living prevention programs

VI. Life Skills
    A. Key concepts: resilience, belonging, mastery, independence, generosity, hardiness
    B. OTA concerns: life skills development, instrumental activities of daily living (IADLs), stress management, relaxation, social skills, assertiveness, anger management, self-concept, goal setting

VII. Activities of Daily Living
    A. Key concepts: occupational performance areas, community living, safety, demonstration, hand over hand, verbal cues, adaptive equipment
    B. OTA concerns: assessment and treatment of grooming, oral hygiene, bathing, toileting devices, dressing, eating, medication, health maintenance, socialization, communication, mobility, emergency response, sexual expression, preparing for sleep

VIII. Work, Play, and Leisure
    A. Key concepts: legislation and regulation, job analysis, work simulation, ergonomics, functional capacity evaluation, graded work tasks, reasonable accommodations, work rehabilitation
    B. OTA concerns: home management, care of others, educational activities, work activities, leisure activities, recreation

MANAGEMENT AND PRACTICE ISSUES

I. Management Issues
    A. Key concepts: accreditation, reimbursement, public relations, service operations, paradigm, fee for service, cost effectiveness, program development, diagnosis-related groups (DRGs), Medicare, quality assurance, AOTA
    B. OTA concerns: record keeping, continuing education, data analysis, inservice training, malpractice, maintaining supplies, *Standards of Practice*, personal credentials

II. Documentation and Reimbursement
    A. Key concepts: confidentiality, patient's rights, third-party reimbursement, prospective payment system, assessment, and discharge note
    B. OTA concerns: facility rules, laws and regulations; *Code of Ethics*; subjective, objective, assessment, plan (SOAP) format; narrative format; goals and objectives

III. Supervision
    A. Key concepts: supervision process, service competence, entry-level practice, regulations and standards
    B. OTA concerns: supervision partnership, supervisor roles, supervisee roles, students, volunteers

IV. Ethics
    A. Key concepts: honesty, truthfulness, morals, *Code of Ethics*
    B. OTA concerns: beneficence (prevent harm), duty (responsibilities), fidelity (keep word), nonmaleficence (do no harm), veracity (be truthful)

V. Team Membership
    A. Key concepts: interdisciplinary, multidisciplinary, transdisciplinary, cross-training, teamwork
    B. OTA concerns: team building develops mastery and maturation

VI. Professional Development
    A. Key concepts: professional socialization, professional development plan, competence
    B. OTA concerns: mentor, life-long learning, skill development

Chapter Four

Fieldwork Experience as a Study Guide

ROLE OF FIELDWORK

The purpose of fieldwork is to integrate classroom study with clinical practice and to develop clinical reasoning skills. To help you use your fieldwork experience to study for the exam, you must first understand some of the policies established by AOTA.

Fieldwork in an accredited OTA school is divided into two types: level one and level two. Level one fieldwork is experienced during your studies, usually done part-time during the academic year. Level two is typically full-time, after you have completed your studies. Of course, due to the shortages of fieldwork sites, your school may have provided you with a creative, nontraditional level-two fieldwork. Although these fieldwork experiences are different from what has been traditional in the past, it is our experience that these students do equally well on the exam.

Much of what you know as an OTA student was developed and refined during your fieldwork experiences. As the NBCOT exam is focused on the "doing" of OT, it is important to use your fieldwork experiences to study. This section of the book is designed to help you review your fieldwork experience. We have provided opportunities to reflect on your areas of accomplishment and those that need further review before you take the exam. Begin by identifying all of your fieldwork sites using the example below.

SAMPLE FIELDWORK REVIEW			
Fieldwork Sites	*Level One*	*Level Two*	*On My Own*
St. Mary's Hospital	Observed hand treatment		Observed peds
Community Mental Health Center		Community skills (IADLs) assessments	
Summer Program for Special Kids			Helped OT run SI groups

Use the following table to identify your fieldwork experiences. Fill in each square with a brief summary of what you did at each fieldwork site. Include both level one and level two fieldwork, and any additional experiences you have had working with an OT.

FIELDWORK REVIEW			
Fieldwork sites	*Level One*	*Level Two*	*On My Own*

Now that you have reviewed your fieldwork experiences, it is time to look at the variety of consumers with which you have worked. Below is a table of diagnostic categories that many OTAs work with. It is not expected that you have had experiences in all these areas. On the contrary, students who focus their experiences in limited areas develop clinical reasoning skills more easily. This table is designed to point out those areas in which you are accomplished and those areas in which you may need to study for the exam. Use a check mark to indicate your assessment of your fieldwork experience. Blank spaces are provided at the end of the table to add other diagnostic categories.

FIELDWORK DIAGNOSIS REVIEW					
Diagnosis	*No Experience*	*Observation Experience*	*Some Experience*	*A Lot Of Experience*	*Community vs Medical Model*
ADHD					
AIDS/Infectious disease					
Amputation					
Anxiety					
Arthritis					
Bipolar disorder					
Blindness					
Burns					
Cancer					
Cardiac disease					
Cerebral palsy					
Child/Elder abuse					
CVA/Neurological issues					
Dementia					
Depression					
Diabetes					

FIELDWORK DIAGNOSIS REVIEW (CONTINUED)					
Diagnosis	No Experience	Observation Experience	Some Experience	A Lot Of Experience	Community vs Medical Model
Drug/alcohol abuse					
Eating disorders					
Hand/arm conditions					
Head injuries					
Learning disabilities					
Low vision/hearing loss					
Mental retardation					
Multiple sclerosis					
Muscular dystrophy					
Orthopedic conditions					
Parkinson's disease					
Personality disorders					
Pervasive developmental disorder					
Schizophrenia					
SI dysfunction					
Spina bifida					
Spinal cord injuries					

After you have completed a review of your fieldwork experiences, it is time to make an assessment of the areas you need to review before the exam. Fieldwork was never intended to provide you with a view of all occupational therapy practice. It would be expected that many of your check marks on the fieldwork diagnosis review table would be in the no experience column.

Setting studying priorities for the exam should begin in the *no experience* and *observation experience* columns. Even with that as a starting place, you may feel like it is too much to manage at once. Use the following chart to set your study priorities.

STUDY PRIORITIES			
Diagnosis	*Top Priority*	*Second Priority*	*No Need to Study*
ADHD			
AIDS/Infectious diseases			
Amputation			
Anxiety			
Arthritis			
Bipolar disorder			
Blindness			
Burns			
Cancer			
Cardiac disease			
Cerebral palsy			
Child/elder abuse			
CVA/Neurological issues			
Dementia			
Depression			
Diabetes			
Drug/alcohol abuse			
Eating disorders			
Hand/arm conditions			
Head injuries			
Learning disabilities			
Low vision/hearing loss			
Mental retardation			
Multiple sclerosis			
Muscular dystrophy			
Orthopedic conditions			
Parkinson's disease			
Personality disorders			
Pervasive developmental disorder			
Schizophrenia			
SI dysfunction			
Spina bifida			
Spinal cord injuries			

Now that you have set your top priorities, consider the amount of time available before the exam and the time you have outside of your current life responsibilities to study. Review Chapter Two of this book and incorporate your priorities in your study plan. Next, review Chapter Three, which outlines study content.

When working on the study questions in the next section, you may find it helpful to think of some of your clients from your affiliations to problem solve the answer to a question. You can organize your study review notes based on classic symptoms versus clinical symptoms you saw on your affiliations. This will allow you to think through a question on the exam with a story visualization of what the patient would look like. Review the example below, then fill out your own table.

CLASSIC VS. CLINICAL PICTURES DURING FIELDWORK (SAMPLE)			
Diagnosis	Patient's First Name	Classic Symptoms	Clinical Symptoms Seen on Fieldwork
CVA—left cortex	Samuel	Expressive aphasia	Mild
		Receptive aphasia	Not present
		Right side weakness	Yes
		Spasticity	Yes, required splint
Schizophrenia	Anna	Withdrawn	No
		Flat affect	Blunted but not flat
		Hallucinations	Heard voices
		Delusions	No
		Poor hygiene	Good with reminder

Use the following table to outline your own patient stories. Fill in the spaces with the classical symptoms based on your class notes and textbooks. Picture the patient in your mind, and fill in the clinical symptoms you saw during your fieldwork.

This exercise will help you answer exam questions using the clinical reasoning skills you developed during fieldwork. When faced with a question such as developing a treatment activity for a person with schizophrenia or a CVA, picture your patient trying each of the available answers. This might help you eliminate wrong answers and zero in on the correct answer.

CLASSIC VS. CLINICAL PICTURES DURING FIELDWORK			
Diagnosis	Patient's First Name	Classic Symptoms	Clinical Symptoms Seen on Fieldwork

CLASSIC VS. CLINICAL PICTURES DURING FIELDWORK (CONTINUED)			
Diagnosis	Patient's First Name	Classic Symptoms	Clinical Symptoms Seen on Fieldwork

SUMMARY

Reviewing your fieldwork experiences will help you recognize both accomplishments and areas that need further study. Examining each diagnosis that you saw during both level one and level two fieldwork will help you to prioritize your studying for the exam. Visualizing patient stories in your mind may help you eliminate wrong answers on the exam and remember correct ones.

SECTION III

Study Questions

Chapter Five

Domain, Task, and Knowledge Questions and Answers

Section One

1. A child with ADHD may show all of the following behavioral limitations *except*:
   A. Poor impulse control
   B. Decreased level of motor activity
   C. Decreased attention span
   D. Poor interpersonal awareness

2. The OTA is treating a child with visual memory problems. Which of the following treatments would *not* be used?
   A. Organizing information into large groups
   B. Using repetition
   C. Using mnemonic devices
   D. Determining differences in stimuli

3. An 82-year-old man is having difficulty seeing. He claims that his sight seems to be clouded, and this problem has been getting progressively worse. What might this condition be?
   A. Glaucoma
   B. Presbyopia
   C. Cataract
   D. Presbycusis

4. Which of the following is *not* a subtype of schizophrenia according to the DSM-IV TR?
   A. Delusional
   B. Paranoid
   C. Disorganized
   D. Catatonic

5. Which of the following reflexes is being demonstrated if a child's head is turned to the left, the left arm and leg are extended, and the right arm and leg are flexed?
   A. Tonic labyrinthine reflex
   B. Positive support reflex
   C. Asymmetrical tonic neck reflex (ATNR)
   D. Symmetrical tonic neck reflex (STNR)

6. Which of the following statements regarding bulimia nervosa is *not* true?
   A. Bulimia is more prevalent than anorexia
   B. Significant weight loss must occur
   C. Self-evaluation is influenced by body shape and weight loss
   D. Recurrent episodes of binge eating occur

7. The final era of life as defined by Eric Erickson is:
   A. Wisdom vs. Senility
   B. Wisdom vs. Faith
   C. Integrity vs. Wisdom
   D. Integrity vs. Despair

8. A patient with a panic disorder with agoraphobia would be treated *most* effectively by?
   A. Cognitive-behavioral treatment
   B. Individual treatment
   C. Group treatment
   D. Family intervention

9. A patient has decreased muscle strength in her right upper extremity (RUE). While sitting, she is asked to raise her arm toward the ceiling. The patient can only raise her arm halfway through range. According to this information, what muscle grade does she have?
   A. Fair
   B. Fair +
   C. Fair -
   D. Poor +

10. Brian is an individual with a traumatic brain injury (TBI) referred to OT. He screams out for no reason and shows aggressive behavior. Verbalization and behaviors are inappropriate and nonpurposeful. His gross attention is short and selective attention is nonexistent. Brian is able to perform self-care given maximum assistance. What RLA level is Brian?
    A. II
    B. III
    C. IV
    D. V

11. Cathy is diagnosed with amyotrophic lateral sclerosis (ALS). During the *first* stage of the disease, occupational therapy should:
    A. Introduce adaptive equipment
    B. Include ROM exercises
    C. Teach breathing exercises
    D. Teach energy conservation

12. Major principles of joint protection techniques include all of the following *except*:
    A. Maintain muscle strength and ROM
    B. Keep joints stable by reducing movements
    C. Reduce forces
    D. Use each joint in the anatomically correct plane

13. An elderly woman is complaining of pain, swelling, and decreased ROM in her hip area. These symptoms *best* describe what following diagnosis?
    A. Osteoporosis
    B. Degenerative bone disease
    C. Hip fracture
    D. Osteoarthritis

14. A patient with difficulty swallowing has:
    A. Dysphagia
    B. Dysarthria
    C. Aphasia
    D. Ataxia

15. Karen is an individual diagnosed with a spinal cord injury (SCI). She is independent with a joystick-operated power wheelchair. What level of SCI usually uses this type of chair?
    A. C5, C6
    B. C7, C8
    C. T1, T2
    D. T3, T4

16. A person recovering from a TBI in an outpatient program requires goals to measure functional improvement. Which of the following are the three components of measurable goals?
    A. Performance, condition, limitation
    B. Data, performance, outcomes
    C. Performance, condition, criterion
    D. Name, occupation, age

17. Standardized tests provide reliable and valid data. To obtain these results, what method should the practitioner use?
    A. Ask any question necessary
    B. Follow the uniform procedures
    C. Follow any procedures as long as all questions are asked
    D. Follow procedure by using layperson terms to gear to the patient

18. What subtype of cerebral palsy involves all four extremities affected with increased muscle tone?
    A. Spastic quadriplegia
    B. Spastic diplegia
    C. Spastic triplegia
    D. Spastic hemiplegia

19. A person has experienced decreased movement in wrist ROM. What is the movement that is performed at the wrist by the flexor carpi ulnaris?
    A. Adduction
    B. Abduction
    C. Flexion
    D. Extension

20. How many pairs of spinal nerves originate from the spinal cord?
    A. 35
    B. 31
    C. 25
    D. 12

21. In a treatment program for a child, tactile stimulation is *best* used when the OTA wishes to perform which of the following?
    A. Enhance the vestibulocochlear system
    B. Stimulate nerve endings
    C. Decrease sensory response
    D. Increase sensory response

22. Following a stroke, an elderly patient has RUE weakness and is unable to feed himself. What is the *best* approach for the OTA to take to address initial feeding?
    A. Stimulate or facilitate the muscle
    B. Guide the arm
    C. Remind the person to use the hemiplegic arm
    D. Encourage feeding tasks

23. A 70-year-old patient has just been diagnosed with Alzheimer's disease. Which of the following is not true of Alzheimer's disease?
    A. Most common form of dementia
    B. Progresses through six stages
    C. Presently has no cure
    D. Always includes memory impairment

24. One of the most significant changes in the elderly population is osteoporosis. Which of the following is *not* a risk factor for osteoporosis?
    A. Obesity
    B. Estrogen depletion in postmenopausal moment
    C. Calcium deficiency
    D. Physical inactivity

25. A child with autism may typically show all of the following motor problems *except*:
    A. Poor physical endurance
    B. Poor gross and fine motor coordination
    C. Delay in response to reflexes
    D. Low tone in extensors and flexors

26. If a child has diminished tendon reflexes and has less than normal resistance to movement, what muscle tone is being demonstrated?

    A. Hyperthermia

    B. Hypotonia

    C. Hypoxia

    D. Intermittent

27. An OTA is running a group in a psychiatric unit when a patient suddenly looks pale and complains of dizziness and shortness of breath (SOB). These symptoms might demonstrate:

    A. Vestibular dysfunction

    B. Generalized anxiety

    C. A panic attack

    D. Delusions

28. Which of the following is *not* one of Mildred Ross' integrative stage groups?

    A. Orientation

    B. Performing

    C. Cognitive stimulation

    D. Closing the session

29. An entry-level OTA with less than 1 year of experience must have close supervision by an OT or advanced OTA. How is close supervision defined?

    A. Constant contact throughout the day

    B. Direct contact once a month with telephone contact as needed

    C. Daily meeting about the treatment sessions

    D. Treating patient together

30. What disorder is characterized by a refusal to maintain body weight, intense fear of gaining weight, and a distorted image of self?

    A. Bulimia

    B. Anorexia

    C. Depression

    D. Self-abuse

31. Which of the following is *most* likely a primary sign of a heart attack?

    A. Headaches

    B. Numbness in the arm

    C. Chest pain or pressure

    D. Hot flashes

32. A patient with a CVA who neglects the paralyzed extremities displays what type of behavior?

    A. Remission

    B. Denial

    C. Anxiety

    D. Forgetfulness

33. A 15-year-old teen has a complete transection of the spinal cord at the T5, T6 level. Before working on transfers, what should be strengthened *first*?
    A. Trapezius
    B. Pectoralis major
    C. Serratus anterior
    D. Latissimus dorsi

34. Dysphasia is caused by:
    A. The incoordination of facial muscles
    B. Sensory loss and muscle weakness of the mouth and throat
    C. Language disorder
    D. Uncoordinated gait

35. Which of the following *best* describes CP?
    A. Cleft spine, which is an incomplete closure in the spinal column
    B. A nonprogressive disorder caused by damage to the central nervous system (CNS), resulting in impaired ability to move efficiently and maintain balance
    C. Uncommon condition detected by genetic testing
    D. Paralysis of arm/hand caused by damage to the limb brachial plexus, resulting in an infant who is large or breech at birth

36. What is the cause of Down syndrome?
    A. Smoking
    B. Alcohol-addicted mother
    C. Chromosomal abnormality
    D. Prematurity

37. When an elderly person has diabetes, what condition can occur with his or her vision?
    A. Macular degeneration
    B. Retinopathy
    C. Glaucoma
    D. Cataracts

38. Which of the following *best* defines AOTA's *Code of Ethics*?
    A. Responsibilities of the OTA
    B. A guide for ethical behavior
    C. Being truthful
    D. All people have the same fundamental rights

39. A teacher at the school system in which you work has been complaining that one of her students is clumsier than the others and also more distracted during class. She says that when she has pictures for the child to look at, the child seems to understand and listen better. What type of problem might this be?
    A. Vestibular processing disorder
    B. Attention deficit disorder
    C. Proprioceptive problem
    D. Tactile defensiveness

40. Within patient documentation, the OTA should:
    A. Write in the third person
    B. Use medical terminology appropriately
    C. Use formal and complete language
    D. All of the above

41. What *best* describes the toe-touch weight-bearing (TTWB) for a total hip replacement (THR) patient?
    A. No body weight is borne on the involved side
    B. Not all of the body weight can be borne on the involved side
    C. No weight-bearing on the heel
    D. Full weight-bearing

42. What *best* describes continuous supervision?
    A. Provided on an as-needed basis
    B. OT supervisor is in sight of the assistant who is performing the client-related task
    C. Direct contact at least every 2 weeks at the site with interim supervision occurring by other methods
    D. Daily direct contact at the site

43. What *best* describes the Mini Mental Status Exam (MMSE)?
    A. Leather lacing tool to assess cognitive level
    B. A series of questions related to cognitive ability
    C. A functional description of performance in ADLs
    D. Twenty-four craft projects analyzed according to the patient's level of cognitive complexity

44. What are the three progressive phases of schizophrenia?
    A. Bipolar, agoraphobia, compulsion
    B. Delirium, vascular dementia, amnesic
    C. Prodromal, active, residual
    D. Catatonic, paranoid, disorganized

45. The Comprehensive Occupational Therapy Evaluation (COTE) scale is a measure of behavior observed during a task. The COTE is:
    A. Nonstandardized
    B. Based on a task using three or more steps
    C. Provides functional descriptions of performance in a variety of ADLs
    D. Both A and B

46. Which of the following activities does *not* involve proprioceptive input?
    A. Hanging from a chin-up bar
    B. Pressing the heel of your hand into clay
    C. Spinning around on a tire swing
    D. Playing tug-of-war

47. Piaget constructed four maturational levels of cognitive function. What level characterizes the shortest but most egocentric thought of mental development?

    A. Sensorimotor

    B. Pre-operational

    C. Concrete operational

    D. Formal operational

48. All of the following are reasons to conduct an evaluation for the purpose of addressing a child's development and functional status *except*:

    A. To determine if the child should be further assessed using comprehensive evaluations

    B. To determine if the child is eligible for occupational therapy services after initial screening

    C. To determine an intervention plan

    D. To evaluate the child in an unfamiliar environment

49. The OTA must be aware of the inability of a fracture to heal properly. All of the following are correct terms that describe a fracture's inability to heal *except*:

    A. Delayed union

    B. Nonunion

    C. Malunion

    D. Midunion

50. An individual that suffers a SCI above the T6 level of the spinal cord with a complete lesion has a greater risk of developing:

    A. Orthostatic hypotension

    B. Brown-Séquard's syndrome

    C. Autonomic dysreflexia

    D. Anterior spinal cord syndrome

Section One Answers and Explanations

1. Answer: B
A high level of motor activity would be a behavioral limitation. Children with ADHD show the symptoms of answers A, C, and D.

2. Answer: A
Answer A is not true because you want to organize information into small units, then progress to a more complex and larger grouping as the child improves. Answers B, C, and D are all good treatments for a child with visual memory problems.

3. Answer: C
Cataract is the clouding of the lens of the eye. The lens increases with age in anterior and posterior diameter as layers of protein develop. The eye becomes more opaque as proteins become increasingly oxidized. Answer A is the loss of the eyes' ability to focus. Answer B is an increase in eye fluids, which causes pressure on the eye and may lead to vision loss. Answer D is the loss of smell.

4. Answer: A
DSM-IV TR classifies subtypes of schizophrenia as paranoid, disorganized, catatonic, undifferentiated, and residual. Answers B, C, and D are true.

5. Answer: C
ATNR is stimulated by the rotation of the child's head. When the head is turned, the reflex causes the arm and leg on the same side as the chin to extend further, while the opposite arm and leg become more flexed. Answers A, B, and D are examples of other reflexes; they do not have the reaction described.

6. Answer: B
According to the DSM-IV TR diagnostic criteria, significant weight loss does not have to occur in order to be diagnosed. Answers A, C, and D are true.

7. Answer: D
Erik Erickson and his colleagues present a view on the changing personality of elders to include the final era of life, integrity vs. despair. Answers A, B, and C are not accurate in describing the final era of life according to Erickson.

8. Answer: A
The two most effective treatments for panic disorder and agoraphobia are pharmacotherapy and cognitive-behavioral therapy. Answers B, C, and D would be less effective treatments.

9. Answer: C
Fair- is when the part of the body moves through incomplete ROM against gravity. Answer A is when the extremity can move through complete ROM against gravity. Answer B is when the extremity can move through complete ROM against gravity with slight resistance. Answer D is when the extremity can move through complete ROM with gravity eliminated.

10. Answer: C
RLA level IV, the confused-agitated level, displays these symptoms. Answers A, B, and D do not show all of these symptoms.

11. Answer: D
In the first stage of the disease, the patient should be taught work simplification and energy conservation techniques because he or she has low endurance and will become tired easily. Answers A, B, and C are not as important but might be considered after answer D.

12. Answer: B

Answer B is correct because you want a patient to avoid staying in one position for long periods of time. Answers A, C, and D are all major principles of joint protection.

13. Answer: D

Osteoarthritis is marked by destruction of joint cartilage leading to exposure and destruction of underlying bone. Because there is a reduction in cartilage, the bones rub together causing inflammation. Inflamed joints are marked by pain, swelling, and decreased ROM. Degenerative bone disease is the same as osteoporosis, which is when the bone becomes porous and deteriorates. Answer C is incorrect because a hip fracture would not become inflamed and swell unless infected or so acute that emergency intervention would be required.

14. Answer: A

Dysphagia is defined as a difficulty with swallowing. Answer B, dysarthria, is having difficulty with speech articulation. Answer C, aphasia, is the inability to produce or understand speech. Answer D, ataxia, is the inability to coordinate the movements of muscles.

15. Answer: B

A person with spinal cord injuries at a level of C7, C8 will be independent with a joystick-operated power wheelchair.

16. Answer: C

Answer C identifies the three necessary components (performance, condition, and criterion) for writing measurable goals. Answers A, B, and D are not likely because they are incomplete and lack the necessary components for writing measurable goals. Other methods (audience, behavior, condition, and degree) are available to write measurable goals. Any practitioner reading the note places the importance on the goals being clear, objective, and measurable.

17. Answer: B

For results to be valid, the practitioner must follow the standardized uniform protocol. Standardized tests have consistent procedures for scoring. The results of an adapted assessment are not valid and reliable.

18. Answer: A

Spastic quadriplegia, also referred to as tetraplegia in SCI, involves all four extremities. Spastic diplegia involves the upper extremities. Spastic triplegia is involvement of three extremities. Spastic hemiplegia is involvement of the extremities on only one side of the body.

19. Answer: C

Flexor carpi ulnaris causes flexion at the wrist. Adduction takes place at the wrist when it is acting with the extensor carpi ulnaris. Abduction is an action that takes place at the wrist when acting with the flexor carpi radialis. Extension of the wrist takes place with the extensor carpi ulnaris.

20. Answer: B

Thirty-one pairs make up the spinal nerves—eight cervical, 12 thoracic, five lumbar, five sacral, and one coccygeal. Answers A, C, and D are not the correct number of pairs of spinal nerves in the spinal cord.

21. Answer: D

Answer D is the best answer because the OTA is treating to increase sensory response. Answers A, B, and C are not the results from performing tactile stimulation on a child, although tactile (deep pressure) and/or vestibular aspects may be used in vestibulocochlear system treatment, stimulating nerve endings, or decreasing sensory response.

22. Answer: B

Guiding the "weak" arm is the best technique to try first. Stimulating or facilitating the muscle is not always the best treatment approach for an elderly patient. Reminding the person to use the hemiplegic arm is possible but not the best approach for an elderly individual. Encouraging feeding tasks is holistic and encouraged throughout treatment sessions.

23. Answer: B

Alzheimer's disease has three stages: mild, moderate, and severe. Answers A, C, and D are all accurate aspects of Alzheimer's disease.

24. Answer: A

Obesity is a risk factor for osteoarthritis. Estrogen depletion in post-menopause, calcium deficiency, and lack of physical activity are important risk factors of osteoporosis.

25. Answer: A

Answer A is a motor problem associated with Down syndrome. Poor gross and fine motor coordination, delayed response to reflex stimulation, and low tone in extensors and flexors are all motor problems exhibited by a child with autism.

26. Answer: B

Hypotonia is defined as decreased muscle tone and less than normal resistance to movement. Hypothermia is low body temperature. Hypoxia is reduced oxygen content in body tissue. Intermittent is occasional and unpredictable resistance to postural changes.

27. Answer: C

Answer C is correct because the stated symptoms are all related to panic attacks. Vestibular dysfunction, although having dizziness and paleness, is characterized by a sensory integration disorder. Generalized anxiety is characterized by nervousness and sweating. Delusions, along with hallucinations and mood disorders, are associated with schizophrenia.

28. Answer: B

Answer B is part of Yalom's group stages. Mildred Ross' stage groups include orientation, movement, visual-motor perceptual activities, cognitive stimulation and function, and closing the session.

29. Answer: C

According to the AOTA guidelines, close supervision is daily, direct contact on site. Routine is defined as direct contact at least every 2 weeks at the site of work. General is defined as monthly direct contact with supervision as needed. Minimal is provided only on an as-needed basis and may be less than monthly.

30. Answer: B

Anorexia is characterized by the symptoms listed. Bulimia is characterized by recurrent episodes of binge eating in which large amounts of food are consumed, followed by self-induced vomiting. Depression is mood affected by agitation, weight loss, and insomnia associated with decreased activity. Self-abuse is afflicting pain upon one's self.

31. Answer: C

Answer C is most likely correct because chest pain or pressure is a sign of a heart attack. Answer A is not as serious as chest pain but may also be seen. Answer B is a sign of a stroke. Answer D can commonly occur to anyone. Caution should be noted as women often do not have chest pain when having a heart attack.

32. Answer: B

Answer B is correct because the patient denies and ignores the paralyzed extremities. Answer A is not correct because remission describes a good state of a disease. Answer C, anxiety, is not part of neglect. Answer D is not correct because the patient appears to be neglecting the paralyzed extremity, and forgetfulness is an unconscious behavior.

33. Answer: D

Answer D is correct. The latissimus dorsi needs to be strengthened because it falls on the T5 and T6 area. The other muscles are not affected at T5 or T6.

34. Answer: B

Answer B is correct because it best describes dysphasia. Answer A defines dysarthria. Answer C relates only to a language issue. Answer D is uncoordinated gait or ataxia.

35. Answer: B
Answer B is correct because it describes CP. Answer A defines spina bifida. Answer C defines Prader-Willi syndrome. Answer D defines Erb's palsy.

36. Answer: C
Down syndrome is caused by a chromosomal abnormality. Answer A does not cause Down syndrome but may cause low birth weight. Answer B causes fetal alcohol syndrome (FAS) in the baby. Answer D can have many causes.

37. Answer: B
Answer B is correct because it occurs when someone is diabetic. Answer A is when the central portion of the retina undergoes deterioration. Answer C occurs in the elderly but is not caused by diabetes. Answer D does not occur from diabetes.

38. Answer: B
Answer B is correct because it defines the *Code of Ethics*. Answer A defines progress notes. Answer C describes veracity, and answer D describes equality, which is part of the *Code of Ethics* but does not define the whole document.

39. Answer: C
Proprioception problems deal with body position being clumsy, awkward, or distracted. Vestibular processing disorders involve the motor functions, such as poor equilibrium and low muscle tone. Symptoms of ADHD include language disabilities, auditory processing, and perceptual impairments. Tactile defensiveness involves a child who would overreact to ordinary touch sensations.

40. Answer: D
Answer D is correct because all of the answers should be in documentation.

41. Answer: C
Toe-touch is no weight-bearing on the heel using the toe for balance. Answer A is no weight-bearing. Answer B describes partial weight-bearing. Answer D is full weight-bearing as the patient can tolerate.

42. Answer: B
Answer B is correct because it describes continuous supervision for the OTA. Answer A is not correct because it describes minimal supervision. Answer C explains routine supervision. Answer D describes close supervision.

43. Answer: B
Answers A, C, and D relate to Claudia Allen's cognitive disabilities frame of reference. Answer A describes a test called Allen's Cognitive Levels (ACL) and cognitive functioning, answer C describes the Routine Task Inventory, and answer D describes the Allen Diagnostic Module.

44. Answer: C
Answer C is correct because they are associated with the phases of schizophrenia. Answer A is cognitive disorders not related to schizophrenia. Answer B is cognitive disorders related to dementia. Answer D is subtypes of schizophrenia. The five subtypes include paranoid, disorganized, catatonic, undifferentiated, and residual type.

45. Answer: D
Answer D is correct because the COTE is nonstandardized and describes behaviors in functional terms. Answer C is not correct because it describes ADL assessments such as the Routine Task Inventory, KELS, or MEDLS.

46. Answer: C
Spinning around on a tire swing employs the vestibular system. Answers A, B, and D are all examples of the muscles and joints informing the brain concerning position of body parts, which are the hallmarks of proprioceptive feedback.

47. Answer: A

According to Piaget, answer A is the period of development characterized by the shortest but most egocentric thought processes. Answer B is incorrect because the pre-operational stage occurs between the ages of 2 and 7 years. During this stage, children learn to alter their environment by using language to access information through organization, serialization, and conservation. Answer C, the concrete operational stage of development, occurs between the ages of 7 and 11. Typically, sensory manipulation and experience drive these children. Answer D addresses the formal operational period of development, which begins at age 11 and focuses on the child's ability to think in more abstract or conceptual terms.

48. Answer: D

It is necessary to place the child in a familiar setting in order to assess the child's functional status. Answers A, B, and C are valid criteria that can be the purpose of conducting an assessment concerning the functional status of a child.

49. Answer: D

Answer D is the one exception that is not a term describing fractures that do not heal. Answer A, delayed union, describes a fracture that heals very slowly. Answer B describes a fracture that stopped healing just before a secure union could form. Answer C describes a bone that does not heal evenly with the remaining bone.

50. Answer: C

Answer C is most likely because individuals who suffer SCIs above the T6 level are more prone to autonomic dysreflexia due to reflex action of the autonomic nervous system. Answer A would not be a good answer because orthostatic hypotension is a sudden decrease in blood pressure. Answer B would not be correct because Brown-Séquard's syndrome results when only one side of the spinal cord is damaged below the level of injury. Answer D is incorrect because anterior spinal cord syndrome results from injury that damages the anterior spinal artery.

Section Two

1. A person with post-traumatic stress disorder and acute stress disorder will be able to deal with his or her problem more effectively if he or she is:
   A. Encouraged to forget what happened and go on with his or her new life
   B. Told feelings of anxiety are normal
   C. Allowed to take sedatives to help relax and engage in activities
   D. Encouraged to express his or her feelings through structured group sessions

2. When assessing the equilibrium and protective reactions of a 5-year-old child with CP, what approach is *best*?
   A. The child should be placed on a bolster
   B. The child should be observed in his or her natural setting
   C. The child should be placed in all appropriate developmental positions
   D. The child should sit on the floor with the trunk supported by the OTA

3. A patient with dysphagia will experience which of the following symptoms?
   A. Difficulty in swallowing
   B. Difficulty in planning and performing motor acts to dress one's self
   C. Sensations such as tingling, numbness, and burning
   D. Restless sleep, irritable mood

4. Presbycusis means "old hearing" and in an elderly person is a:
   A. Buzzing, ringing, whistling, or roaring in the ears that is most noticeable at night
   B. Type of high-frequency hearing loss
   C. Type of low-frequency hearing loss
   D. Period of deafness

5. A 23-year-old individual was recently in a car accident that caused an injury to the left side of her brain. Which of the following activities would be *best* suited for her treatment sessions?
   A. Drawing
   B. Checkers
   C. Bicycle riding
   D. Jigsaw puzzles

6. An OTA is leading a group on body image for persons with anorexia nervosa. Which of the following would be the *best* activity to do within the group?
   A. Woodworking
   B. Magazine collage
   C. Ceramics
   D. Nutritional pyramid

7. A 5-year-old boy with developmental delays and poor frustration tolerance is unable to don or doff his winter jacket independently. What treatment approach would be *best*?
   A. Provide the child with a zipper pull
   B. Use backward chaining
   C. Use forward chaining
   D. Suggest the purchase of a pullover jacket

8. Which of the following is the *most* effective method of donning a button shirt for a person with left hemiplegia?

   A. Dress the left arm first, then the right arm

   B. Dress the right arm first, then the left arm

   C. Button the shirt first, and use the over-head method

   D. Use a button hook

9. Mary is a 69-year-old female with impaired vision. She is experiencing difficulty viewing the television to watch the morning news. Which of the following would be the *most* appropriate suggestion to make?

   A. Move the television toward a window

   B. Move the television away from any windows

   C. Use red or orange strips of tape to mark the buttons on the remote control

   D. Purchase a large-screen TV

10. The OTA is leading a small group when a client with a history of drug abuse strikes out at another member. Which of the following is the *first* thing the OTA should do?

    A. Attempt to overpower and restrain the client

    B. Call for more staff

    C. Talk to the client to calm him or her down

    D. Ask the other group members to ignore the negative behavior in order to prevent negative reinforcement

11. The OTA is leading a group of four newly admitted women with major depression in an inpatient psychiatric facility. During the first session, which of the following would be the *best* approach?

    A. Allow the patients to choose one activity from a choice of five or six

    B. Choose an activity that requires sustained attention for 30 to 45 minutes

    C. Choose a craft activity that requires quick responses, thereby keeping the patients focused on the task

    D. Choose simple, structured short-term activities

12. A mother has reported that in the morning before school her child becomes angry and throws a tantrum during their normal routine, especially during dressing. Which of the following might the child be demonstrating?

    A. Tactile defensiveness

    B. Over-anxious disorder

    C. Proprioception problems

    D. Oppositional defiant disorder

13. A person with a severe burn in the latter stages of hospitalization experiences increased localized and severe pain at the mid-range of elbow flexion. Which of the following conditions should the OTA suspect?

    A. Orthostatic hypertension

    B. Humeral fracture

    C. Heterotopic ossification

    D. Ulnar nerve injury

14. Following a left CVA, Joe, a 67-year-old retired assembly worker, is being treated by OT. Joe complains of pain and stiffness in his left hand while completing a woodworking activity. Which of the following conditions might the OTA suspect?

    A. Osteoarthritis

    B. Heterotopic ossification

    C. Osteoporosis

    D. Contractures

15. An OTA observes an OT treating a male patient who has had a CVA. The therapist encourages the patient to use both sides of the body during treatment activities and facilitates slow, controlled movements. What treatment approach is the OT *most* likely using?

    A. NDT

    B. Biomechanical approach

    C. Proprioceptive facilitation

    D. Sensory integration

16. Which of the following is *not* a common side effect of antipsychotic drugs?

    A. Photosensitivity

    B. Extrapyramidal symptoms

    C. Postural hypotension

    D. Continuous drowsiness

17. At 3 years of age, self-feeding consists of the following *except*:

    A. Little or no spilling

    B. Holding a fork in the fingers without sliding

    C. Drinking from a cup with one hand

    D. Pouring from a light pitcher into a cup if the pitcher is not too heavy

18. At what RLA level is it *most* appropriate for a person with a TBI to drive again?

    A. VI

    B. VII

    C. X

    D. It is never appropriate for a person with a TBI to return to driving

19. Mary, a 77-year-old female, is experiencing aphasia following a stroke. What facilitation of communication techniques would be *most* appropriate for the therapist to provide Mary's family?

    A. Speak loudly, and make sure Mary is able to see the person speaking

    B. If Mary does not respond immediately to a question, repeat the question

    C. Always use "yes" and "no" questions when conversing with Mary

    D. Use gestures when speaking to Mary

20. Which of the following statements about the ADA is *not* true?

    A. An employer is required to make reasonable accommodations unless doing so would create significant difficulty or expense, as determined by specific guidelines

    B. A business may be allowed to provide home delivery instead of remodeling its building to accommodate people with disabilities

    C. Private clubs are required to be accessible to people with disabilities

    D. An employer may refuse to hire someone who poses a significant risk to the health and safety of other employees

21. Which of the following groups statistically have the higher percentage of people who attempt or commit suicide?
    A. People who have a terminal illness
    B. People who have been diagnosed with a mental disorder
    C. People who are within the ages of 18 to 25
    D. People who have recently lost a significant other

22. All of the following describe symptoms of spastic quadriplegia in a child with CP *except*:
    A. Mental retardation often occurs
    B. The mouth and tongue are affected
    C. There is wide cerebral dysfunction
    D. The legs are clearly more affected than the arms

23. When preparing the patient for a transfer out of bed, what should the OTA do *first*?
    A. Explain what you expect from the patient during the transfer
    B. Place a gait belt around the patient when he or she is sitting at the edge of the bed
    C. Position and lock the wheelchair, then move the leg rests out of the way
    D. Have the patient move forward to the edge of the bed or chair

24. Which is *not* a principle of joint protection?
    A. Use the strongest joints available for the activity
    B. Avoid positions of deformity
    C. Ask a family member to assist with task performance
    D. Avoid using muscles or holding joints in one position for any length of time

25. Prior to an out-of-bed transfer during an ADL session, you notice that the patient with a recent total hip replacement (THR) has a calf that is warm to the touch, painful, and red. The *best* action to take is:
    A. Complete the ADL, then notify the nurse
    B. Ask nursing for pain medication for the patient
    C. Inform nursing and keep the patient in bed until further instructions are received
    D. Apply an ice pack on the leg for 15 minutes, then complete the ADL session

26. What type of onset has a *better* prognosis for a person diagnosed with schizophrenia?
    A. Onset acute and late in life
    B. Onset insidious and early in life
    C. Onset acute and early in life
    D. Onset insidious and late in life

27. A child with brain damage has neurological impairment, motor deficits in development, and an impaired ability to maintain normal postures due to lack of normal muscle tone. What condition might be present?
    A. Cerebral palsy
    B. Muscular dystrophy
    C. Epilepsy
    D. Tonic-clonic seizures

28. During the initial dip of the client's hand into the paraffin bath, the client withdraws her hand and states it is too hot. The patient does *not* have any sensory or cognitive issues including past trauma with heat. Skin is intact. How do you proceed after checking the temperature and setting, which is 125°F?

    A. Reschedule treatment and allow the paraffin to cool down, then complete treatment

    B. Discontinue treatment and call the maintenance department

    C. Reassure the client and continue treatment

    D. Discontinue treatment and consult with an OT

29. Which of the following is the *best* method for a stand-to-sit transfer technique when working with a person who has had a THR?

    A. Extend the operated leg forward, reach back for arm rests, and slowly sit down, being careful not to lean forward at the hips

    B. Reach back for the arm rests, allow the patient to sit quickly in the chair, being careful not to lean forward

    C. Have the patient look back and reach for the arm rests, lean back, and slowly sit down in the chair

    D. Reach back for the arm rests, extend the operated leg forward, and slide the non-affected foot forward

30. A stroke patient who has difficulty determining the distance between the observer and objects, figures, or landmarks, in addition to having difficulty with changes in planes of surfaces, exhibits what perceptual processing problem?

    A. Position in space

    B. Depth perception

    C. Spatial relations

    D. Figure ground

31. After a chart review, the OTA enters the patient's room for an ADL session. The individual is an 80-year-old man who underwent a THR. He is disoriented to place and time with a decreased attention span. The chart stated the patient is "A and Ox3." The patient might be exhibiting symptoms of what cognitive disturbance?

    A. Delirium

    B. Dementia

    C. Hallucination

    D. Psychotic episode

32. A child has a hearing problem. His mother states that when she speaks to her son loudly he seems to be able to hear her. When she speaks to him in a normal tone, he reacts like she is standing far away. Which of the following is this hearing disorder characteristic of?

    A. Low tone loss

    B. Deafness

    C. Flat loss

    D. High tone loss

33. After completing yesterday's independent exercise program of moist heat and active range of motion (AROM), a patient with rheumatoid arthritis (RA) states that she felt pain in her joints for 30 minutes after. What is the *best* treatment for today's session?

    A. Moist heat and passive range of motion (PROM) only

    B. Moist heat and the same exercise program

    C. Ice area and PROM only

    D. Ice and immobilize affected joints in splint

34. In RA, what primary area of the body is *most* affected?
    A. Hands
    B. Tendons
    C. Synovial joints
    D. Ligamentous tissue

35. An OTA is alone in the department and catching up on paperwork in a long-term care facility after hours. Nursing calls for a wrist splint per MD order for a patient who just fell. What is the *best* plan of action according to the AOTA *Standards of Practice*?
    A. Check for the MD order for the splint, measure the wrist, and place a splint with stockinet as directed in the facility protocol
    B. Call the OT at home and have her instruct you on how to proceed
    C. Supply the nurse with the splint to don on the patient
    D. Notify the staff that you will schedule the patient to be seen by an OT first thing in the morning

36. A patient was just admitted to your facility with a recent onset of symptoms, including decreased energy level, loss of appetite and weight, changes in sleep and activity level, and problems making decisions. These symptoms are characteristic of which one of the following disorders?
    A. Major depression
    B. Dysthymic disorder
    C. Anorexia
    D. General anxiety disorder

37. When given a pencil, a child holds it horizontally and squeezes it so tightly that his knuckles turn white. What type of grasp is this?
    A. Precision grasp
    B. Power grasp
    C. Hook grasp
    D. Cylindrical grasp

38. What is the *best* occupational therapy treatment for trigger finger?
    A. AROM to strengthen the flexor digitorum superficialis
    B. Moist heat to the palm to improve tissue mobility, and use ice to decrease inflammation of the area
    C. Splint the affected finger for a few days to immobilize the joint
    D. Paraffin treatment to the affected hand, then AROM to the painful joints

39. A patient comes into your facility with a THR. She complains that she has a habit of dropping things, such as clothes and her pocketbook. Her husband is tired of picking up after her and says he will not do it any more. Which of the following should you suggest?
    A. Tell her to bend over and pick it up herself; it is allowed
    B. Tell her husband that he needs to help her for at least 6 weeks until she can do it herself
    C. Suggest she purchase a reacher with an extended handle so she can pick up things independently
    D. Advise her to sit in a chair and pick the objects up off the floor

40. The intermediate-level OTA is able to supervise:
    A. Aides, technicians, entry-level OTAs, volunteers
    B. Aides, technicians, entry-level OTAs, volunteers, level I OT fieldwork students, level I and level II OTA fieldwork students
    C. Aides, technicians, entry-level OTAs, volunteers, level I OT fieldwork students, and level I OTA field work students
    D. Aides, technicians, volunteers

41. As a treatment activity, you have your patient with Bipolar I disorder perform a magazine picture collage. When reviewing the collage, you notice that the patient has placed large cuttings on the paper. Which of the following likely describes this form of expression?
    A. Grandiosity
    B. Hostility
    C. Passion
    D. Security

42. Which list of characteristics *best* describes Prader-Willi Syndrome (PWS)?
    A. Children are obese, short in stature, and have decreased muscle tone, a long face, and slanted eyes
    B. The syndrome causes a child to be tall and thin
    C. Most often affects boys
    D. Children have one additional chromosome

43. While performing an activity of daily living treatment with a patient who had a stroke, you notice that the patient is having trouble dressing. The patient proceeds to put his left sleeve on the right arm. The patient then becomes frustrated with the activity and insists on not wearing the shirt. What is the *best* explanation for the problem?
    A. The patient has unilateral neglect
    B. The patient has a low frustration level
    C. The patient has a body scheme disorder
    D. The patient has apraxia

44. Which of the following is *not* a form of physical restraint?
    A. Posies
    B. Wheelchair tray
    C. Recliner
    D. Valium

45. During a treatment session, your patient confides in you that she is afraid of a certified nursing assistant (CNA) on the unit. She states that the CNA treats her roughly, is rude, and does not allow her to select her own clothing each day. As a professional, what is your *first* responsibility in this situation?
    A. Talk to the CNA directly about the patient's concerns
    B. Report the incident to the head nurse on the unit
    C. Talk to administration about the patient's comments
    D. Report the incident to your supervisor

46. The following are characteristics of negative symptoms in schizophrenia *except*:
    A. Lack of emotional responses
    B. Social withdrawal
    C. Poverty of speech
    D. Auditory hallucinations

47. According to AOTA, a fieldwork coordinator at a college or university must obtain what qualifications?
    A. Three years of practice experience
    B. Experience in supervision of fieldwork students
    C. Experience advising fieldwork students
    D. All of the above

48. You assist a SCI patient with a supine-to-sit transfer after some mat work. The patient immediately complains of dizziness and nausea while in the sitting position. What is the OTA's *best* approach?
    A. Tell the patient to hold on while you finish the transfer
    B. Remove restrictive clothing after seating the patient
    C. Have the patient sit in place until the nausea subsides
    D. Stop the transfer and recline the patient quickly

49. On a home evaluation of a person with a THR with a history of falls, you notice that when she is walking around her home she is very hesitant. When you ask her about it, she says she is afraid of falling again. What is making her feel this way?
    A. Biological issues
    B. Psychosocial issues
    C. Functional issues
    D. Environmental issues

50. What AOTA document stipulates that an occupational therapy practitioner shall respect the recipient and/or their surrogate(s), as well as the recipient's rights?
    A. *Occupational Therapy Standards of Practice*
    B. *Occupational Therapy Practice Framework*
    C. *Occupational Therapy Philosophy*
    D. *Occupational Therapy Code of Ethics*

Section Two Answers and Explanations

1. Answer: D

Answer D is most correct because it is important for the patient to express his or her feelings. Answers A, B, and C are incorrect because they allow the patient to avoid the problem and do not teach coping strategies.

2. Answer: C

Reactions occur in all developmental positions (i.e., supine, prone, quadruped, kneeling, standing). Answers A and D are less likely because these positions may not necessarily address all the positions that need to be observed. Answer B is less likely because the child may not use all developmental positions while being observed in his or her natural setting.

3. Answer: A

Answer A is most correct. B is the definition of dressing apraxia. C is the definition of paresthesia. D is an example of dyssomnia, a sleep disorder.

4. Answer: B

Answer B lists the symptoms of presbycusis. Answer A lists symptoms of tinnitus. Answer C is incorrect because low-frequency sounds are more readily heard. Answer D is incorrect because presbycusis is not characterized by periods of deafness.

5. Answer: D

Answer D is the best answer because it involves an activity that requires the patient to pay more attention to detail and spatial relationships. Answer A is incorrect because drawing requires minimal scanning. Although checkers (answer B) does require scanning, it does not require attention to detail or comparison of objects. Answer C is incorrect because the activity does not focus on the primary cognitive issues being addressed.

6. Answer: B

Magazine picture collages allow expression of personality and self. Answers A and C are less likely because they typically allow for less expression of one's body image. Answer D is less likely because it is not a task used for the expression of body image. It would be more applicable to a nutritional group.

7. Answer: B

The child will receive positive reinforcement by completing the task, providing the child with immediate success. Answer C, forward chaining, is less likely because it does not provide immediate success and may increase frustration. Answers A and D are less likely because they may not address the area of difficulty in donning the jacket (i.e., sequencing, body awareness). Also, answers A and D require the caregiver to purchase an item and teach compensation without first using a remedial approach.

8. Answer: A

The affected arm should be dressed first. In this case, the left arm is the affected arm; therefore, answer B is not correct. Answer C is not likely because front button shirts are typically easier to don. Answer D is not correct because it does not address donning the shirt.

9. Answer: B

Glare-producing objects, such as the television, should not be placed near light sources. Answer A is less likely because moving the television toward the window may increase glare. Answer C is less likely because it does not address Mary's ability to view the television. Answer D is less likely because other treatment recommendations should be made before suggesting the purchase of a new item.

10. Answer: B

Calling for additional staff should be the first step when this situation occurs. Answer A is incorrect because the OTA should never attempt to overpower the client. Answers C and D are less likely because after calling for additional staff, the other clients should be removed from the area, then staff can attempt to calm the client down.

11. Answer: D

The activity is simple and allows for success. Answer A is not effective because decision-making abilities may be impaired. Answer B is not likely because the patients may have decreased attention span; therefore, short-term activities should be used. Answer C is not effective because activities requiring rapid movements should be avoided.

12. Answer: A

Tactile defensiveness involves the tendency to overreact to ordinary touch sensations. These responses can include anger, tantrums, aggression, and emotional distress. Answer B is incorrect because over-anxious disorder involves extreme self-consciousness, excessive and unrealistic worries, and anxiety about competence. These feelings were not noted. Answer C is incorrect because proprioception problems include problems with the muscles and joints informing the brain about position of the body parts. Answer D is incorrect because oppositional defiant disorder includes the child blaming others for his or her own actions, which the child has not done.

13. Answer: C

Heterotopic ossification is a complication associated with burns and is characterized by the symptoms stated. Answer A is not correct because orthostatic hypertension is not characterized by the symptoms provided in the case. Answer B is incorrect because fractures are not typically associated with severe burns. Answer D is incorrect because ulnar nerve injury typically results in a sensory loss on the ulnar side of the hand.

14. Answer: A

The symptoms presented are characteristic of osteoarthritis, and Joe has a work history in which repetitive actions are likely to have caused damage to the joints in his hands. Answer C is incorrect because the symptoms presented do not correspond to those of osteoporosis. Answers B and D are incorrect because the left hand was not affected by the CVA.

15. Answer: A

Incorporating both the affected side and unaffected side of the body, along with using slow, controlled movements, are both characteristics of NDT. Answers B, C, and D are incorrect because they do not incorporate the treatment methods described.

16. Answer: D

Continuous drowsiness is not a common side effect of antipsychotic drugs, although initial drowsiness may be present. The other symptoms may be present; therefore, answers A, B, and C are true.

17. Answer: B

Holding a fork appears at age 4 and older. Answers A, C, and D are functional tasks typically developed by age 3.

18. Answer: C

At stage X, judgment has returned and persons are typically independent. Answer A is incorrect because at stage VI persons are still dependent on external input. Answer B is incorrect because at stage VII the person lacks insight on his or her condition and demonstrates decreased judgment and problem solving. Answer D is incorrect because many persons who have had TBIs recover and return to driving.

19. Answer: D

Demonstration and gestures can help convey information. Answer A is incorrect because it is not appropriate to speak loudly to someone with aphasia. Answer B is incorrect because adequate time should be given to allow Mary to respond. Answer C is incorrect because using yes and no questions exclusively would limit communication and is likely below Mary's communication abilities.

20. Answer: C

Private clubs are not required to be accessible; however, they may choose to make their facilities accessible. Answer A is true of the ADA. Answer B is true because the ADA allows for alternate ways of providing goods and services if barriers cannot be removed. Answer D is true because an employer may refuse to hire someone if there is a significant risk established based on reliable medical evidence.

21. Answer: B

Ninety-five percent of all people who commit or attempt suicide have a diagnosed mental disorder, although they may not be receiving mental health services. Answers A, C, and D are incorrect—suicide rates increase with age. The rate for those 75 and older is more than three times the rate among young people.

22. Answer: D

Answer D is not true because the arms (flexors) are more affected than the legs (extensors) in spastic diplegia. Answers A, B, and C are characteristic of spastic quadriplegia.

23. Answer: C

It is especially unsafe to look for or reach for the chair after the patient is already sitting up in bed. Answer A is an important point; however, the ending point of the transfer should be in place during discussion of transfer for visual cues to assist with patient comprehension of the transfer activity. Also, when supine, the patient cannot easily see the environment and equipment to be used during the transfer. Answer B is also an important point; however, the OTA should discuss the transfer and gait belt prior to use. Answer D is incorrect because for safety reasons the wheelchair should be in place before the patient sits at the edge of the bed.

24. Answer: C

Typically, the patient is encouraged to use adaptive equipment or alternate methods prior to asking for assistance to promote independence with activities. Answers A, B, and D are all appropriate principles of joint protection.

25. Answer: C

These symptoms are consistent with those of a deep vein thrombosis (DVT). A DVT, especially one located below the knee, may become loose and pass to the lungs, producing a pulmonary embolism. The patient should not move from the bed until the doctor or nurse rules out DVT.

26. Answer: A

Prognosis is best with late, acute onset.

27. Answer: A

The question describes symptoms of cerebral palsy. Answers B, C, and D are incorrect. Muscular dystrophy is not a neurological condition; it is characterized by muscle wasting. Epilepsy and tonic-clonic seizures are not likely because they typically do not interfere with normal development.

28. Answer: C

The paraffin temperature for treatment is 125° to 130°F. Answers A, B, and D are incorrect. There is no need to reschedule treatment because the temperature is at the low end of the acceptable level. The patient may be reluctant on initial trial of paraffin due to unfamiliarity of the process.

29. Answer: A

Answer A is more likely because the person must reach back for the armrests and slowly sit down without leaning forward. Answer B is not correct because the person should never sit down quickly into a chair. Answer C is not correct because having the patient look back might cause him or her to lose balance or bend the hip. Answer D is incorrect because having both feet slide forward will cause the hip to bend forward and the person to quickly sit down in the chair.

30. Answer: B

The given definition relates to depth perception. Position in space involves relationship of figures and objects to self or other objects. Spatial relations involve position of objects relative to each other. Figure ground involves differentiating between foreground and background forms and objects.

31. Answer: A

Forty to fifty percent of all patients recovering from hip surgery have an episode of delirium. Answer B is a possible answer in relation to a somatic cause or medication induced; however, dementia typically develops over time. The mental status change of this particular patient is rapid and related to the surgery time. Hallucinations and a psychotic episode may seem an appropriate issue, but delirium is most common in this type of surgery. Hallucinations and psychotic episodes better describe schizophrenia.

32. Answer: C

All frequencies are evenly affected by flat loss. When the client is near the source, noises and voices sound far off in the distance. Answers A, B, and D are incorrect. Low and high tone loss do not make the sound seem far off in the distance. They are characterized by sound detection of vowels and consonants. Deafness would be loss of the ability to hear.

33. Answer: B

Pain lasting one or more hours is a signal to change current activity. Answers A, C, and D are not appropriate because stated complaints of pain do not indicate a negative physical response to the exercise program.

34. Answer: C

The synovial joints break down first in the disease process. Answers A, B, and D are incorrect because they are secondary complications to the synovial joint breakdown.

35. Answer: D

According to Standard II: Referral, an OT must evaluate the patient prior to treatment. Answer A is incorrect because an OTA cannot evaluate the patient or don a splint without OT instruction. Answer B is incorrect because it is not appropriate to call the OT at home for this situation, unless the facility has an on-call policy. Answer C is incorrect. The OTA would need to determine the type and size of the splint to be issued to nursing.

36. Answer: A

Answer A is correct because these are characteristics of major depression. Answer B is incorrect because dysthymic disorder is a chronic disorder characterized by the presence of a depressed mood for most of the day, whereas major depression is characterized by episodes. Although answer C consists of changes in sleep activity, appetite, and weight, a person may not have trouble making decisions. Answer D is less likely because there is no decrease in energy level in most cases.

37. Answer: B

When using the power grip, the pencil is horizontally held and squeezed tightly. Answer A is incorrect because the precision grasp requires a light grasp and opposition of the fingertips to hold an object. Answer C is incorrect because a hook grasp does not utilize the thumb and is typically used to hold heavy objects. Answer D, cylindrical grasp, is used for larger objects, such as a drinking glass. The fingers are not as flexed during this grasp.

38. Answer: C

Immobilization of the joint allows the FDS tendon to rest. Answers A and D are unlikely because trigger finger is not a muscle problem. It is best to avoid joint movement that increases irritation of the FDS tendon. Answer B is a valid treatment, however, but not the best because it would not provide the longest lasting benefit. Answer D is not recommended because it is best to avoid joint movement that increases irritation of the FDS tendon.

39. Answer: C

The extended reacher will help her to pick up the objects she drops and increase her sense of independence, while maintaining THR precautions. Answers A and D are incorrect because they do not follow THR precautions. Answer B is not likely because occupational therapy focuses on increasing independence and reducing the caregiver's role when possible.

40. Answer: B

The intermediate-level OTA is able to supervise aides, technicians, entry-level OTAs, volunteers, level I OT fieldwork students, and level I and II OTA fieldwork students. Answers A, C, and D are incorrect according to the AOTA guidelines.

41. Answer: A

The large pictures represent thinking in a grand way. Answer B is less likely because hostility is more associated with thick lines on the paper. Answer C is less likely because passion is associated with red paper. Answer D is less likely because security is associated with green paper.

42. Answer: A

Children with PWS are typically obese, short in stature, have decreased muscle tone, a long face, and slanted eyes. PWS is also associated with a defect in chromosome 15. Answer B describes Klinefelter's syndrome. Answer C describes neurofibromatosis, which is more common in boys. Answer D describes characteristics of Down syndrome.

43. Answer: C

Answer C is most likely because the issue is the person placing the left sleeve on the right arm. Answer A is not likely because the person acknowledges the other side of the body. Answer B is not likely because the low frustration level is due to the inability to put on the shirt. Answer D is not likely because the person has the motor planning ability to put the shirt sleeve on the arm.

44. Answer: D

Valium is a chemical restraint. Answers A, B, and C are physical restraints.

45. Answer: D

Principle 7 of the *Code of Ethics* requires the OTA to report the incident to the "appropriate authorities." Her supervisor would be the first person with whom she would discuss the situation. Answers A, B, and C may be implemented after the OT is informed; however, the OT should be notified first.

46. Answer: D

Auditory hallucinations, although common in schizophrenia, are a positive symptom. Positive and negative symptoms are ways to classify the behaviors that occur in schizophrenia. Negative symptoms describe the characteristics that are absent, while positive symptoms describe the symptoms that are productive or present.

47. Answer: D

According to AOTA, a person must obtain all of these qualifications in order to work as an academic fieldwork coordinator. Answers A, B, and C are all required qualifications.

48. Answer: D

Answer D is most important because the patient is showing signs of a dangerous situation, known as orthostatic hypotension. The transfer should not continue, and the patient should sit back down and be reclined quickly. Answer A is not likely because the patient could pass out while in the middle of the transfer. Answer B is not likely because the patient is still sitting up and is medically unstable. Answer C is not likely because the person has not been reclined and is still in the upright position.

49. Answer: B

Poor judgment, fear of falling, and fatigue make up this cause; however, the OTA should probe for additional biological, functional, or environmental issues.

50. Answer: D

Answer D is the correct answer. The *Code of Ethics* addresses autonomy, privacy, and confidentiality of the patient. Answers A, B, and C are AOTA documents; however, they do not address the above statement. The *Standards of Practice* defines the occupational therapy process. *Practice Framework* provides a consistent terminology base for health care professionals, and the *Philosophy of Occupational Therapy* makes no specific statements regarding patient rights; it explains the mission of occupational therapy.

Section Three

1. What is the *next* step in the assessment process after the referral is made, the screening has been completed, and the evaluation has been finished?
   A. Discharge summary
   B. Plan treatment
   C. Develop goals
   D. Begin treatment interventions

2. The OTA's role in splinting would *most* likely be:
   A. Construct static and dynamic hand splints independently
   B. Evaluate the longevity and necessity of the splint, as well as review the proper handling and care of the splint
   C. Construct and adjust the splints, and educate the patient/family on use and care under supervision of the OT
   D. Clean and maintain the area that is going to be splinted

3. What type of treatment would you recommend for a child suffering from tactile discrimination problems?
   A. Sensory integration (SI) therapy
   B. NDT treatment
   C. Cognitive developmental treatment
   D. Proprioceptive neuromuscular facilitation (PNF) treatment

4. The hook grasp is used:
   A. To hold the handle of a briefcase
   B. To hold onto a key
   C. To write with a pen
   D. To pick up a basketball

5. An OTA is required to have close supervision by an OT when:
   A. The patient's condition is acute, complicated, and rapidly changing
   B. Dressing and grooming are involved
   C. Using a checklist to gather a patient's general history
   D. Any type of treatment plan is being carried out

6. A C7-level SCI often results in:
   A. COPD
   B. Monoplegia
   C. Paraplegia
   D. Tetraplegia

7. OTAs working in the school system can:
   A. Provide direct service to children under the supervision of an OT
   B. Complete an initial evaluation and SOAP note each week
   C. Work with children without the supervision of an OT; however, only in the school setting
   D. Teach any elementary school grade as long as there are children with disabilities present

8. What is *not* a common chronic disease of aging?
   A. Cancer
   B. Osteoporosis
   C. Hypertension
   D. Guillain-Barré syndrome

9. A primary purpose for the OTA when working with the elderly is:
   A. To help them explore leisure activities
   B. To search for a new place of employment because they have trouble finding one on their own due to their age
   C. To develop toileting and medication schedules
   D. To restore function so they can return to completing the tasks they were able to do before injury or decline

10. Which of the following characteristics is commonly seen with the diagnosis of delirium?
    A. Lack of orientation
    B. Coherent speech
    C. Slow onset of symptoms
    D. Sequenced thinking

11. In order for an OTA to treat a child with CP:
    A. The OT must be confident in the OTA's knowledge, experience, and educational background, which must surpass the usual assistant-level educational background
    B. The OTA must have parental approval
    C. Minimal experience is needed, such as general knowledge of abnormal tone and at least one previous fieldwork experience in a pediatric setting
    D. This is not possible; OTAs do not treat children with CP

12. What are the three leading causes of death for people 65 years and older?
    A. Schizophrenia, diabetes mellitus, Guillain-Barré syndrome
    B. Heart disease, cancer, CVA
    C. Diabetes mellitus, cancer, Alzheimer's disease
    D. Heart disease, CVA, diabetes mellitus

13. Major depression is:
    A. Most commonly seen in children
    B. A mood disorder
    C. A personality trait that cannot be changed
    D. A problem when an individual is grieving over a death for more than 1 week

14. The OTA's role in treating a geriatric patient is:
    A. To complete a screening and evaluation to determine problematic areas
    B. To supervise staff in providing recreation and socialization activities, along with supervising any type of psychological treatments
    C. Provide treatment, such as to increase or restore muscle strength, joint mobility, and coordination given supervision or consultation from an OT
    D. To decide on adaptive equipment and take appropriate measurements for wheelchairs and walkers

15. Which of the following is *not* a mental health disorder?
    A. Bulimia
    B. Autism
    C. TBI
    D. Depression

16. The OTA is working with a child with ataxic CP who is experiencing decreased muscle tone in the head and trunk. Which of the following gentle treatments would you select?
    A. Rocking
    B. Shaking
    C. Bouncing
    D. Speaking with a calm voice

17. Your patient is a 14-year-old girl who has anorexia nervosa. What performance component is the *most* important to focus on in treatment?
    A. Feeding and eating
    B. Self-concept
    C. Self-expression
    D. Health maintenance

18. What is the lowest level an OTA must reach to supervise OT aides, technicians, care extenders, volunteers, level I OT fieldwork students, and level I and II OTA fieldwork students?
    A. Entry level
    B. Intermediate level
    C. Advanced level
    D. Never

Use the following information to answer questions 19 and 20:

Bob is recovering from a TBI. He is inconsistently oriented to time and place. He can follow simple one-step directions consistently. He shows decreased ability to process information. Bob has increased his awareness of self, family, and basic needs, but short-term memory (STM) is impaired.

19. According to the RLA scale of cognitive functioning, at what level is Bob?
    A. RLA IV, confused-agitated
    B. RLA V, confused, inappropriate, non-agitated
    C. RLA VI, confused-appropriate
    D. RLA VII, automatic-appropriate

20. Which of the following is the *most* appropriate treatment for Bob?
    A. Give him a list of directions for tasks
    B. Work on problem solving with him
    C. Help him keep a memory logbook
    D. Have him make a collage of family photos

21. What is the *most* important factor to consider regarding developmental milestones in children?
    A. The sequence
    B. Chronological age
    C. Reaching physiological milestones prior to psychosocial milestones
    D. Reaching cognitive milestones prior to physiological milestones

22. Mrs. Jenkins is a 65-year-old woman who suffers from RA in both upper extremities (BUE). She is currently suffering from an acute-stage flare-up. What is the *best* treatment exercise to maintain joint mobility?
    A. AROM with slight stretch at end range
    B. PROM with slight stretch at end range
    C. AROM to the point of pain
    D. PROM to the point of pain

23. You are scheduled to treat Mr. Johnson, who has been diagnosed with AIDS. On your way to his room, your coworker stops and asks you to see her patient, Mrs. Smith (who has had a THR), because she has to go pick up her daughter at school. When you explain that you are scheduled to see Mr. Jones, she says, "He can wait. He is not going to get better anyway, and Mrs. Smith is so sweet and loves therapy." According to the AOTA *Code of Ethics*, what following principle *best* addresses this situation?
    A. Beneficence/autonomy
    B. Competence
    C. Compliance with laws and regulations
    D. Public information

24. Your patient with schizophrenia says to you, "Some people have a hard time believing that I have been alive for 2,000 years, but I have." This is an example of what?
    A. An illusion
    B. Delirium
    C. A delusion
    D. A hallucination

25. Your 35-year-old patient has been in trouble with the law since he was 15 years old. He has been arrested for stealing and assault several times. He is aggressive toward others in therapy group and has been caught lying to several members on more than one occasion. When confronted by one of the group members who caught him lying, he showed no remorse. What disorder does he *most* likely have?
    A. Paranoid personality disorder
    B. Antisocial personality disorder
    C. Histrionic personality disorder
    D. Borderline personality disorder

26. You are working with a child who has severe oral-sensory defensiveness. Which of the following foods would you attempt to introduce *first*?
    A. Ice cream
    B. Oatmeal
    C. Mashed bananas
    D. Plain yogurt

27. Your patient suffered a severe CVA and has experienced a prolonged period of bed rest. When you try to get her out of bed, you notice her right lower extremity (RLE) is warm to touch. The patient complains of tenderness when you touch it. You uncover the leg, and it appears red. You suspect:

    A. Autonomic dysreflexia

    B. Hemiplegia in RLE

    C. Pulmonary embolus

    D. DVT

28. You are working on dressing with a patient with Alzheimer's disease. He is having trouble with attention span, body awareness, sequencing, and ability to follow directions. What is the *best* technique to use with this patient?

    A. Use 100% cotton clothing, since it does not retain the odor of urine

    B. Use verbal and visual cues to simplify each step

    C. Have the patient use a reacher to pull his pants on over his feet

    D. Have the patient identify safety hazards in the bathroom and bedroom

29. According to the AOTA, all of the following key performance areas are within the scope of practice for an OTA with intermediate skills *except*:

    A. Schedules and prioritizes own workload

    B. Participates in fieldwork education process under the direction of an OT

    C. Selects, adapts, and implements intervention under the supervision of an OT

    D. Contributes to program planning and development in collaboration with an OT

30. Which of the following answers is *true* about geriatric sexuality?

    A. Impotence is not a natural consequence of aging

    B. Elders are often too tired to engage in sexual activity

    C. Many older people are too frail to engage in sexual activity

    D. Most elders are no longer interested in sex

31. A patient comes into a therapy session with an affected left side due to a CVA. You notice he has slight edema in his left leg, and you know he has a past history of DVT. What is the *first* recommendation you would make to the patient after checking with his doctor?

    A. Start an exercise program

    B. Remain in bed until the edema is no longer present; do exercises in bed

    C. Get out of bed as soon as possible

    D. Get out of bed as soon as possible, and position legs below heart level

32. A child comes into therapy with a diagnosis of vestibular insecurity. The *most* helpful thing to do in the therapy session would be to:

    A. Have the child remain connected to surfaces as much as possible

    B. Have the child remain disconnected with surfaces at all times

    C. Place the child on a swing to help him or her relax

    D. Have the child ride a bike to practice balancing

33. A child is having difficulty swallowing, and intervention is needed. When treating this child, the most important issue would be:
    A. Creating a bond with the child
    B. Choosing food that is the child's favorite
    C. Making sure the child is seated in the proper position
    D. Nutrition and weight gain

34. Intervention is needed for feeding a child. When is the *best* time to do this?
    A. When the child appears to be hungry
    B. Lunch time
    C. Snack time
    D. During playtime when the child is relaxed

35. Intervention is needed for a child with motor planning problems. During observation you would watch for:
    A. The child's motor control when coloring
    B. The child's ability to change directions in movement
    C. The child's ability to bring both hands together in front of the body
    D. How the child releases with one hand and the need for support on a surface

36. Fluid intelligence relates to:
    A. Memory loss
    B. Alzheimer's disease
    C. Biology, process of aging
    D. Experiences throughout one's life

37. The main purpose of a resting hand splint is to:
    A. Reduce edema
    B. Relieve pain due to subluxation
    C. Maintain the hand in a functional position
    D. Rest the hand when there is a flare-up

38. What would the OTA expect to see in a patient with Parkinson's disease?
    A. Festinating gait, pill rolling, and slurred speech
    B. Festinating gait, pill rolling, and emotional lability
    C. Pill rolling, slurred speech, and repetitiveness
    D. Emotional liability, resting tremors, and festinating gait

39. When a patient has the right triceps graded F- (3-), a short-term goal would be:
    A. Improve strength to F (3)
    B. Improve strength to F+ (3+)
    C. Improve strength to G- (4-)
    D. Improve strength to G+ (4+)

40. A static hand splint should hold the wrist in the:
    A. Functional position
    B. Flexion position
    C. Anatomical position
    D. Position of rest

41. What technique is *not* correct when addressing energy conservation with a patient who tires easily?
    A. Sit for as many activities as possible
    B. Keep items in their familiar locations
    C. Use a bridging technique during home management activities
    D. Bathe or shower at the time of day when you have the most energy

42. What type of supervision is characterized by direct, on-site contact at least every 2 weeks with other contacts, such as telephone or email, used as needed?
    A. General supervision
    B. Close supervision
    C. Continuous supervision
    D. Routine supervision

43. What is the *first* healing stage of bone repair?
    A. Callus formation
    B. Hematoma
    C. Remodeling
    D. Recanalization

44. What are the four symptoms a patient would exhibit in order to be diagnosed as having a manic episode?
    A. Distractibility, sleep disturbances, racing thoughts, and grandiose behavior
    B. Grandiose behavior, hallucinations, increased activity level, and distractibility
    C. Delusions, distractibility, sleep disturbances, and increased activity level
    D. Guilt, talkative, distractibility, and increased inactivity level

45. In order to increase resistance while hammering, one could:
    A. Use fewer nails
    B. Use harder wood
    C. Use larger nails and a heavier hammer
    D. Both B and C

46. Which of the following series of letters are high-frequency sounds?
    A. Z, T, F
    B. S, G, Z
    C. T, F, S
    D. All of the above

47. If a patient complains of blurred vision all the time, especially when he or she sees car headlights, what would the OTA *most* likely suspect?
    A. Glaucoma
    B. Cataracts
    C. Diabetic retinopathy
    D. Macular degeneration

48. In what order does swallowing occur?
    A. Oral phase, oral preparatory phase, pharyngeal phase, esophageal phase
    B. Oral preparatory phase, pharyngeal, oral phase, esophageal phase
    C. Oral preparatory phase, esophageal phase, oral phase, pharyngeal phase
    D. Oral preparatory phase, oral phase, pharyngeal phase, esophageal phase

49. What is Axis II on the DSM-IV TR?
    A. Global assessment
    B. Clinical conditions
    C. Personality disorders
    D. Psychosocial functioning

50. Todd is a 46-year-old man who has an inability to recognize familiar objects. What do you suspect he has?
    A. Apraxia
    B. Angina
    C. Aphasia
    D. Agnosia

Section Three Answers and Explanations

1. Answer: C

Answer C is the next step because the goals must be implemented before the treatment is planned or carried out. A discharge summary is not a possible answer because the patient will still be in need of services. Answer B is not likely because there must be specific goals that the therapist and patient make together before beginning to plan treatment. Treatment interventions cannot be done because the treatment plan has not been developed.

2. Answer: C

If the OT feels that the OTA is competent in this area, he or she can carry out this treatment supervised. Answer A is not likely because OTAs need to be supervised and directed by the OT in order to construct a splint. Answer B is unlikely because an OTA cannot evaluate this independently. Answer D is incorrect because, even though OTAs may be able to perform the preparation, answer C is the best answer.

3. Answer: A

SI therapy is often used with children that have tactile discrimination problems. Answer B is unlikely because NDT therapy is usually used on individuals with hemiplegia who have suffered from a CVA. Answer C is a cognitive treatment that is often used in pediatrics, however, not for tactile discrimination problems. Answer D is used for the population with mostly motor problems.

4. Answer: A

A handle requires a hook grasp. A key requires a lateral pinch. A pen requires a pinch grasp. A basketball requires a full hand grasp.

5. Answer: A

There is the potential for a serious situation in which the OT may need to assist in treatment in answer A. An entry-level OTA is competent in carrying out ADLs. Answer C is unlikely because, if needed, the OT can look over the checklist at a later time. The OTA may carry out treatments with patients in areas in which they show competency.

6. Answer: D

A C7 SCI is a high-level injury resulting in tetraplegia, where the individual will suffer full body paralysis. Answer A is unlikely because COPD is a lung condition unrelated to a SCI. Monoplegia is unlikely because it means one extremity is affected. Paraplegia is unlikely because this means only the lower extremities are affected.

7. Answer: A

OTAs are allowed to provide direct service when supervised by an OT, as long as competence has been demonstrated. OTs are responsible for the evaluation process; however, OTAs may assist. SOAP notes are not done in the school systems; progress notes are done instead. Answer C is unlikely because the OTA is not allowed to practice without supervision. Answer D is unlikely because an elementary school certification is required in order to teach.

8. Answer: D

Guillain-Barré syndrome is an autoimmune disease with no known cause and is not related to aging. Answers A, B, and C are all chronic diseases associated with aging.

9. Answer: D

An OT practitioner's scope of practice is to help increase independence and to restore function. Answer A is also correct but is not a primary concern. Answer B is unlikely because most of the elderly who are receiving OT services are retired. Answer C is unlikely because not all elderly people need a schedule, and, if need be, the OT is responsible for implementing one.

10. Answer: A

Orientation is one of the main issues with delirium and includes incoherent speech. Answer C is not likely because delirium has a rapid onset of symptoms. Answer D is not likely because disorganized thinking is prevalent with delirium.

11. Answer: A

An OTA working in a site that services children with CP is likely to have the necessary skills. The supervising OT has the final responsibility for treatment. Parental permission is always required to treat a child in occupational therapy. The OTA may or may not need specific permission, depending upon the state and facility rules. Answer C is unlikely because this disorder is difficult to treat and more than general knowledge is needed. Answer D is unlikely because OTAs, after gaining enough experience, can treat children suffering from CP.

12. Answer: B

Heart disease, cancer, and CVA are the three leading causes of death of those age 65 and older.

13. Answer: B

Major depression is considered a mood disorder. Children are not the most common age group seen with this type of depression, whereas those 18 and older are more commonly affected. Depression is unlikely because this is not always a personality trait and is treatable. Answer D is unlikely because this falls within a normal length of time to grieve over a death.

14. Answer: C

OTAs can provide treatment related to performance components and areas under the supervision of the OT. Answer A is unlikely because the OT is required to participate in the evaluation and screening process. Answer B is unlikely because OTAs do not supervise psychological treatments. Answer D is incorrect because the OT makes the recommendation about adaptive equipment and sometimes takes wheelchair measurements depending upon the facility.

15. Answer: C

TBI is not specifically a psychiatric diagnosis, although mental health disorders may be secondary to the TBI. Bulimia, autism, and depression are all classified as mental health disorders in the DSM-IV.

16. Answer: C

Gentle bouncing helps to increase muscle tone in the head and trunk. Answers A, B, and D are not likely because these are all methods used to decrease muscle tone.

17. Answer: B

People with this disorder have trouble with self-concept, which leads to self-denying food. Answers A and D are not performance components but are performance areas that may be incorporated into treatment. Answer C is not the most important but may be used as a way of developing a healthy self-expression.

18. Answer: B

According to the AOTA *Guide for Supervision of Occupational Therapy Personnel*, answer B is most appropriate. The entry-level OTA cannot supervise fieldwork students. Answer C is not the lowest level. Answer D is not correct.

19. Answer: C

His ability/impairment is consistent with that of RLA VI, confused-appropriate. Answers A and B are unlikely because he has increased awareness of self, family, and basic needs, which is not typically characteristic of lower levels on the RLA scale. Answer D is unlikely because he is still inconsistently oriented to time and place.

20. Answer: C

Answer C is most likely because he has decreased STM, which will contribute to other problems with function. Working on this area will help with several areas of difficulty he is having. Answer A is not likely because he can only follow one-step commands. Answer B is not likely because he has the inability to process information. Answer D is not likely because he has increased awareness of family and self.

21. Answer: A

It is more important that a child reach the milestones in proper sequence (e.g., crawls before walking) to develop the necessary skills for proper development of the next milestone. Answer B is not likely because children develop milestones at varied ages. Development is not linear; it is a continuous process, and physiological development occurs simultaneously with cognitive and psychosocial development.

22. Answer: C

The goal of OT is to encourage independence. In an acute-stage flare-up, stretch at end of range is contraindicated as suggested in answers A and B. Answer D is not likely because the therapist does the PROM, not the patient. Also, it is always best if the patient can do AROM.

23. Answer: A

According to the AOTA *Code of Ethics*, beneficence/autonomy states that OT personnel shall demonstrate a concern for the welfare and dignity of the recipient of their services. The individual is also responsible for providing services without regard to race, creed, national origin, sex, age, handicap, disease entity, social status, financial status, or religious affiliation. This coworker is discriminating against Mr. Jones because of his diagnosis. Answer B is not likely because the principle of competence states that OT personnel shall actively maintain high standards of professional competence. While this principle could fit, it focuses more on education, skill, and knowledge. Compliance with the laws and regulations may also be broken here, but it is not the best answer for addressing this problem. Public information principle states that OT personnel shall provide accurate information concerning OT services.

24. Answer: C

A delusion is a false belief. An illusion is a belief based on misinterpretation of external stimuli. Delirium is a disoriented reaction associated with fear and hallucinations. A hallucination is a false sensory perception not associated with real, external stimuli.

25. Answer: B

According to the DSM-IV TR, the criteria for a diagnosis of antisocial personality disorder includes the previously mentioned symptoms, such as a failure to conform to social norms with respect to lawful behaviors as indicated by repeatedly performing acts that are grounds for arrest; deceitfulness, as indicated by repeated lying, use of aliases, or conning others for personal profit or pleasure; aggressiveness, as indicated by repeated physical fights or assaults; and lack of remorse. Answers A, C, and D are not likely because the symptoms this patient has do not match the criteria for these personality disorders, according to the DSM-IV TR.

26. Answer: D

Puréed smooth foods are the first solid foods to attempt with a child with severe oral-sensory defensiveness. Answers A, B, and D come after puréed smooth foods (C is the next progression, then B, then A).

27. Answer: D

The symptoms mentioned are symptoms of a DVT, which is common after prolonged periods of immobility and after a CVA. This can be a medical emergency and requires that treatment be stopped immediately. Answer A is not likely because it is a common precaution associated with SCI. Answer B is not likely because it is a paralysis common after CVA but is not associated with these symptoms. Answer C is not likely because it involves the lungs, not the lower extremity (LE).

28. Answer: B

The patient is having trouble with sequencing and following directions. Answer A is a suggestion for incontinence problems. He does not necessarily need a reacher, and equipment may further confuse him. Answer D is not appropriate for dressing but for safety, which cannot be addressed at this point.

29. Answer: D

According to AOTA official documents, the OTA must have high-proficiency skills to be able to perform program planning and development. Answers A, B, and C are all within the scope of practice for an OTA with intermediate skills according to the official documents.

30. Answer: A

Answer A is most likely because impotence is a result of a specific problem and does not happen in all elderly men. Answers B, C, and D are common myths about geriatric sexuality and are untrue.

31. Answer: C

Answer C is the first recommendation you would make because getting out of bed and using the leg is helpful in preventing edema and possible blood clots. Answers A and B are not likely because the patient needs to get out of bed as soon as possible and remain active to help reduce blood clots and edema. Answer D is not likely because the legs need to be positioned above heart level.

32. Answer: A

Answer A is most likely because a child with vestibular insecurities needs to be connected with a surface (typically the floor) at all times. Answers B, C, and D would be unlikely because the child is not connected with surfaces.

33. Answer: C

Proper positioning will increase safety while eating. Bonding, favorite foods, nutrition, and weight gain are also important but are addressed after safety.

34. Answer: C

Snack time is a time when all the children will be eating, but it is not as important as lunchtime should the experience be uncomfortable. Answer A would be unlikely because the child may appear to be hungry but is not. Answer B is less likely because you do not want the child to relate the experience with lunchtime if the experience is unpleasant. It could increase the problem. Answer D is unlikely because you do not want to single out one child in the group. Also, the other children playing could be distracted by the food.

35. Answer: B

Answer B would be the most likely answer because it directly involves motor planning; however, answers A, C, and D could provide additional understanding of the problem.

36. Answer: C

Fluid intelligence relates to skills acquired through incidental learning. Answer A is not related to fluid intelligence. Answer B is unlikely because Alzheimer's is a disease in which the memory is impaired. Answer D is not likely because it relates to crystallized intelligence.

37. Answer: C

A resting hand splint will maintain the hand in a functional position. Answers A, B, and D are unlikely because edema, subluxation, and rest are not the purpose of a resting hand splint.

38. Answer: A

Answer A would be most likely because these are all symptoms of Parkinson's disease. Answers B and D would be unlikely because emotional lability is not a symptom. Answer C would be unlikely because repetitiveness is not a symptom.

39. Answer: A

Answer A would be most likely because that would be the next step up. Answers B, C, and D would be unlikely because they are too much of an increase for a short-term goal.

40. Answer: A

The OTA will want to keep the hand in a functional position. Answers B, C, and D would be unlikely because you would not want to have the hand maintained in any of those positions.

41. Answer: B

It is recommended that items be rearranged according to their frequency of use. Answers A, C, and D are all correct energy conservation techniques.

42. Answer: D

Routine supervision requires direct contact at least every 2 weeks at the site with interim contact occurring by other methods. General supervision is at least monthly direct contact with supervisor and other methods as needed. Close supervision is daily direct contact at the site. Continuous supervision is when the OT is in sight of the aide who is performing delegated client-related tasks.

43. Answer: A

Callus formation is the first step in the healing process. Answers B, C, and D are unlikely because they follow callus formation.

44. Answer: A

Answer A would be most likely because these are all symptoms of a manic episode. Answers B and C would be unlikely because hallucinations and delusions are symptoms of schizophrenia or mood disorders with psychotic features. Answer D would be unlikely because guilt is a symptom of major depression.

45. Answer: D

Answer D would be most likely because these adjustments would make the task more difficult. Answer A is wrong because fewer nails would make the task too easy.

46. Answer: D

The letters Z, T, F, G, and S are all high-frequency sounds (e.g., doorbells and telephones).

47. Answer: B

Cataracts are a filmy coating on top of the eye that causes blurring and halos around lights. Glaucoma is caused by damage to the optic nerve, diabetic retinopathy is caused by damage to the retina, and macular degeneration is caused by damage to the macula.

48. Answer: D

The correct order is oral preparatory phase, oral phase, pharyngeal phase, esophageal phase.

49. Answer: C

Axis I has the clinical psychiatric conditions, Axis II has the personality disorders, Axis III has the general medical conditions, Axis IV has the environmental and psychosocial functioning, and Axis V has the global assessment.

50. Answer: D

Apraxia is the inability to perform motor behavior, angina is a choking pain, and aphasia is a disturbance of language use.

Section Four

1. When treating a child with sensory processing problems, what problem should be assessed and addressed *first*?
   A. Sensory defensiveness
   B. Sensory registration
   C. Sensory integration
   D. Sensory modulation

2. You are a new graduate OTA who has been treating a stroke patient. During treatment sessions, you notice that the patient has difficulty swallowing, as well as trouble with speech at times. You mention this fact to your supervising OT, who asks you to make a referral to speech therapy. What do you do?
   A. Comply with the OT's request and refer the patient to speech therapy
   B. Ask the OT to supervise the referral process because you have not done it before
   C. Ask the OT to make the referral because, as a new graduate, you are not allowed to refer patients
   D. Inform the OT that OTAs are not allowed to make this type of referral

3. A person with a right CVA resulting in left homonymous hemianopsia would have the *most* difficulty seeing objects in which of the following visual fields?
   A. Nasal side of the left eye
   B. Temporal side of the left eye
   C. Temporal side of the right eye
   D. Temporal and nasal sides of the right eye

4. A recreational therapist in the skilled nursing facility (SNF) at which you work asks you to make some recommendations concerning an 82-year-old patient in her recreation group. He has decreased fine motor skills, and the recreational therapist suspects he will have difficulty using the scissors and glue to complete their next project—a magazine picture collage. What do you suggest?
   A. The patient should skip the next group and attend one at which he will be more successful
   B. Adapt the activity by providing glue sticks and self-opening scissors
   C. Show the recreational therapist how to use hand-over-hand techniques to help the patient cut and glue his collage
   D. Make a splint for the patient

5. Which of the following is *not* a sign of aspiration?
   A. Coughing while eating or drinking
   B. Nausea while eating or drinking
   C. Throat clearing while eating or drinking
   D. Wet vocal quality while eating or drinking

6. A 32-year-old man diagnosed with bipolar disorder, whom you have been treating, tells you that he has been thinking about suicide. Which of the following should be your *first* response?
   A. Assure the patient that he is depressed right now, but things will get better
   B. Ask the patient why he wants to commit suicide
   C. Ask the patient if he has a plan
   D. Tell the patient he should talk to a counselor about his thoughts

7. Which of the following statements is *not* true about attention and aging?
    A. Elderly people have more difficulty switching attention between complex tasks
    B. The ability to sustain attention on one task declines significantly with age
    C. It is more difficult to filter out or block background distractions with age
    D. Attention switching declines with age

8. A child with vestibular dysfunction may exhibit which of the following difficulties during functional activities?
    A. Difficulty changing head position to use the sink and mirror in the same task
    B. Lack of balance while feeding
    C. Disorientation when bending over the sink
    D. Difficulty keeping place on the page during reading tasks

9. According to AOTA *Practice Framework*, which of the following is not an IADL?
    A. Socialization
    B. Home management
    C. Care of others
    D. Meal preparation/clean-up

10. Which of the following cognitive techniques would *not* be part of a behavioral training program for clients with mental health disorders?
    A. Thought blocking
    B. Flooding
    C. Assertiveness training
    D. Desensitization

11. Which of the following is *not* a risk factor for Alzheimer's disease?
    A. Female gender
    B. Alcohol abuse
    C. First-degree family history
    D. History of head injury

12. Which one of the following feeding problems is characteristic of autism or PDD?
    A. Fetishes about food
    B. Oral-motor planning problems
    C. Hypertonia
    D. Primitive sucking and swallowing

13. Cognitive impairments in the elderly are believed to be caused by which of the following?
    A. Disease
    B. Aging
    C. Disuse
    D. All of the above

14. John is a 45-year-old man who was involved in a car accident. He is currently at RLA level V. Which of the following *best* describes the goal of treatment for John's current level?
    A. Managing agitation
    B. Providing appropriate stimulation
    C. Maximizing independence
    D. Managing confusion

15. The client you are working with demonstrates the following signs and symptoms: anorexia, insomnia, and fatigue. These are all physiological indications of disturbances that might be associated with:
    A. Mood
    B. Affect
    C. Perception
    D. Insight

16. While working with a SCI patient, you decide to move the patient from supine to an upright position. The patient becomes dizzy, nauseous, and has a loss of consciousness. What is the *first* thing you should do?
    A. Recline the patient quickly
    B. Loosen his or her clothing
    C. Call nursing
    D. Check to make sure the catheter does not have an obstruction

17. Your SCI patient complains of a pounding headache, anxiety, perspiration, chills, nasal congestion, and bradycardia. What is the *first* thing you should do?
    A. Recline the patient quickly
    B. Loosen all restrictive clothing
    C. Check the leg bag tubing for obstruction
    D. Place the patient in an upright position

18. All of the following are precautions to be followed after a THR *except:*
    A. No trunk flexion past 90 degrees
    B. Do not internally rotate legs
    C. Sit on a low surface
    D. Do not lie down without supporting the leg with a pillow

19. Hemiplegia is defined as the loss of sensorimotor function of what?
    A. Both limbs on one side of the body
    B. Both limbs on both sides of the body
    C. Just the lower extremities
    D. Just the upper extremities

20. Tetraplegia is defined as partial or complete paralysis of what?
    A. Upper extremities
    B. Lower extremities
    C. Upper and lower extremities
    D. Both limbs on one side of the body

21. All of the following are examples of an anxiety disorder *except*:
    A. Agoraphobia
    B. Social phobia
    C. Panic attacks
    D. Delirium

22. This disorder is distinguished by physical symptoms, suggesting a medical condition, yet the symptoms are not fully explained by the medical condition, by substance use, or by another mental disorder. Which of the following disorders *best* fits this description?
    A. Somatoform disorder
    B. Anxiety disorder
    C. Obsessive-compulsive disorder
    D. Schizophrenia

23. What neurotransmitter is *most* recognized with schizophrenia?
    A. Dopamine
    B. Serotonin
    C. Norepinephrine
    D. Amino acids

24. All of the following are examples of a developmental disability *except*:
    A. Mental retardation
    B. Cerebral palsy
    C. Autism
    D. Sensory defensiveness

25. Which of the following is *not* an activity used to increase the level of arousal in children?
    A. Sit and spin
    B. Bouncing on a person's lap
    C. Outdoor swings
    D. Rocking slowly on someone's lap or in a rocker chair

26. To increase hand strength for gripping and handwriting, all would be appropriate activities *except*:
    A. Playing with resistive materials, such as clay, dough, or putty
    B. Hammering nails into a board
    C. Encouraging the child to wring out sponges and dishcloths
    D. Have the child place his or her hands in wet oatmeal and leave them there for a short time

27. When an Alzheimer's patient has decreased self-care skills (ADLs), which of the following would *not* be a potential solution?
    A. Simplify clothing/environment
    B. Without nagging, gently encourage the person to do as much as possible
    C. Offer supervision
    D. Dress the person yourself

28. According to G.P. Mulley, what is a more positive term for retirement?
    A. Leisure
    B. Dependence
    C. Fourth age
    D. Third age

29. Which of the following visual skills is *not* shown to decline with advancing age?
    A. Visual processing speed
    B. Light sensitivity or ability to see well in dim light
    C. Color vision
    D. Near vision, especially problematic for reading small print

30. As an entry-level OTA, what type of supervision is required?
    A. General supervision
    B. Routine supervision
    C. Close supervision
    D. Not required

31. All of the following are true about the role of an OTA *except*:
    A. The OTA can carry out parts of the patient screening process under OT supervision
    B. The OTA may select appropriate evaluation instruments in order to administer an evaluation to the patient
    C. The OTA can contribute to the treatment plan
    D. The OTA can educate physicians and other potential referral sources about how to initiate occupational therapy referrals

32. What would be the *most* appropriate response for a therapist to use when trying to establish a therapeutic relationship with a patient who is upset?
    A. Give the patient advice
    B. Relate what the patient has said to one's own experience, so the patient can see that you understand him or her
    C. Offer the patient reassurance
    D. Actively listen to the patient

33. Proper body alignment is necessary for all the following reasons *except*:
    A. Normalization of tone
    B. Preparation for movement
    C. Increased comfort level
    D. Prevention of deformity

34. Which of the following sections would *not* be included on an initial evaluation report?
    A. Treatment progress section
    B. Clinical evaluation section
    C. General information section
    D. Functional status evaluation section

35. As the OTA working with an individual with Parkinson's disease, what treatment goal would you *not* focus on?

A. Prevention of contractures and deformities

B. Increase endurance

C. Maintain or increase strength and ROM

D. Increase level of productivity in ADLs

36. Which of the following problems is *not* generally seen after a person has a CVA?

A. Auditory deficits

B. Tactile deficits

C. Perceptual deficits

D. Motor impairments

37. When treating an upset child with tactile defensiveness, which of the following is the *best* way to approach and touch the child?

A. Approach the child from the side and apply firm pressure on the shoulder

B. Approach the child from behind and apply light touch

C. Approach the child from the front and apply light touch

D. Approach the child from the front and apply firm pressure

38. As the OTA working with a 70-year-old woman with a THR, which of the following hip precautions should the patient follow?

A. No adduction, limited extension, and no external rotation

B. No adduction, limited flexion, and no external rotation

C. No adduction, limited flexion, and no internal rotation

D. No abduction, limited extension, and no internal rotation

39. Which of the following would you use to help a patient in the beginning stage of Alzheimer's disease perform ADLs?

A. Use specific step-by-step instructions during the activity

B. Provide the patient with written instructions on how to complete the activity

C. Structure the environment and cue the patient during the activity

D. Encourage the patient to try to perform as much of the routine as he can on his own

40. What is the prominent symptom of a panic attack?

A. Extreme perspiration

B. Extreme fear and a sense of death or doom

C. Rapid heart rate and nausea

D. Fainting

41. When working with an elderly person with RA, which of the following treatment goals should *not* be a focus during treatment activities?

A. Increase strength

B. Decrease pain and inflammation

C. Preserve function

D. Prevent deformity

42. Which of the following is *not* a clinical feature of post-traumatic stress disorder (PTSD)?
    A. A pattern of avoidance and emotional numbing
    B. The re-experiencing of an event
    C. Fairly constant hyperarousal
    D. Episodes of extreme manic behavior

43. As the OTA doing an initial observation of a child in a school-based setting, what should be your *main* focus of attention?
    A. Review written documents, such as information in the student's file and referral notes
    B. Administration of a standard screening tool
    C. Talk to the teacher and other school personnel about perceived functional problems the child may be experiencing
    D. Observe the child during performance of functional activities in the educational environment

44. Which of the following would you *not* focus on while working with a child with handwriting problems?
    A. Legibility
    B. Grade level
    C. Writing speed
    D. Ergonomic factors

45. What is the cause of schizophrenia?
    A. Increased level of chemicals in the brain
    B. Lesions on the brain
    C. Social stresses
    D. Unknown

46. Who developed the cognitive levels that grade patients on a scale from 1.0 to 6.0 based on their cognitive status?
    A. Claudia K. Allen
    B. Ann Cronin Mosey
    C. Lorna Jean King
    D. Gary Kielhofner

47. In a THR, which of the following precautions is *always* observed?
    A. Use TTWB
    B. Patient cannot bear weight
    C. Patient cannot flex hip greater than 90 degrees
    D. Patient should keep legs at external rotation as much as possible

48. While treating a patient with ALS, he complains of difficulty picking up objects and performing fine motor tasks. What is the treatment priority?
    A. Work on maintaining strength in the extremities
    B. Talk to him about his disease process
    C. Work on maneuvering with a wheelchair and using a reacher
    D. Maintain the ROM, especially in the shoulders and elbows

49. When working with a person with autism, what is *not* a typical behavior?
    A. Lack of awareness
    B. Delayed or abnormal development
    C. Impairment in communication
    D. Easily distracted by new activities

50. What is an infant's first method of mobility?
    A. Standing
    B. Creeping
    C. Rolling
    D. Sitting

Section Four Answers and Explanations

1. Answer: A

Answer A is the best choice because the individual needs to be able to tolerate input without triggering the fight/flight/fright response before registration, integration, and modulation of sensory stimuli can be addressed.

2. Answer: D

According to AOTA *Standards of Practice*, OTs are responsible for making referrals. OTAs are not involved in this process.

3. Answer: B

Homonymous hemianopsia results in loss of the visual field in the corresponding right or left half of each eye. Lesion of the optic tract, after the fibers have crossed at the optic chiasm, accounts for the visual deficit being in the left half of the eye following a right CVA.

4. Answer: B

Providing adapted equipment to allow the patient to be as independent as possible is the best answer. All activities should be made accessible to patients, and grading of the activity can be done so that the patient can participate in the collage. The recreational therapist is not trained to use specific techniques, such as hand-over-hand. Also, hand-over-hand techniques are more appropriate for dyspraxia. A splint would not help the patient increase his fine motor skills.

5. Answer: B

Coughing, throat clearing, and wet vocal quality are all indications of possible aspiration. Nausea is not a recognized symptom of swallowing dysfunction.

6. Answer: C

Answer C is the best choice because the OTA should determine how serious the patient is about suicide. It also provides the opportunity to discuss issues openly. Answer A is incorrect because the OTA should not patronize or placate the patient. Answer B is incorrect because the question "why" is guilt-inducing. Answer D is not appropriate as the first step because the OTA should deal with the patient's statement and not simply refer him to someone else.

7. Answer: B

Answer B is the best choice because sustained attention has been shown to suffer mild to no decline with age.

8. Answer: C

Answer C is the best choice because maintaining orientation while moving requires use of the vestibular sense. Answer A is an example of proprioceptive dysfunction, B is a balance issue, and D is a visual processing problem.

9. Answer: A

Answer A is the correct choice because it is under Social Participation in the official *Practice Framework* document. Choices B, C, and D are IADLs according to *Practice Framework*.

10. Answer: C

Behavioral techniques focus on developing the patient's cognitive skills through education, so answers A, B, and D are appropriate for a behavioral training program. Assertiveness training is not a behavioral technique, so choice C is the best answer.

11. Answer: B

Female gender and a history of either head injury or family diagnosis are both risk factors. Alcohol abuse is not specifically related to Alzheimer's disease, although it does play a role in other cognitive disabilities.

12. Answer: A

Children with autism or PDD will often only eat certain foods, displaying pickiness or fetishes. Answer B applies to children with sensory processing dysfunction, and answers C and D to those with cerebral palsy.

13. Answer: D
Many theorists now believe that disease, aging, and disuse impact cognition in the elderly.

14. Answer: D
RLA level V corresponds to confused-inappropriate-nonagitated behavior. Answer A is more appropriate for RLA level IV, answer B most suitable for RLA levels I to III, and answer C more applicable to RLA levels VII to X.

15. Answer: A
Variations in eating, sleeping, and energy are all possible indications of mood disturbances.

16. Answer: A
Answer A is the first step because with lack of muscle tone in the abdomen and LE pooling of blood can occur, which results in a decrease in blood pressure. Answers B, C, and D are steps that you would take if your patient was experiencing autonomic dysreflexia.

17. Answer: D
Answer D is the first step because the patient is experiencing autonomic dysreflexia. Answers B and C are appropriate *after* sitting the patient up because you should then loosen all restrictive clothing, check the leg bag tubing for obstruction, and call nursing. Answer A is incorrect because this is appropriate for orthostatic hypotension.

18. Answer: C
A THR patient is instructed to not sit on low surfaces because this typically causes the hips to flex beyond 90 degrees. Answers A, B, and D are all precautions of a THR.

19. Answer: A
A patient is described as having a right hemiplegia when both upper and lower right extremities are affected.

20. Answer: C
A patient is described as having tetraplegia when both left and right upper and lower extremities are affected, although the person may have some use of the UE. Answer B is called paraplegia, and answer D is called hemiplegia. Answer A, only UE, would not result from a SCI but is possible from an injury such as a knife wound in the back but not on the spinal cord.

21. Answer: D
A, B, and C are all examples of an anxiety disorder. Answer D, delirium, is characterized by a disturbance of consciousness and a change in cognition that develops over a short period of time.

22. Answer: A
Somatoform disorder is characterized by many somatic symptoms that cannot be explained adequately on the basis of physical and laboratory examinations.

23. Answer: A
Dopamine is the neurotransmitter that has received the most attention with schizophrenia. The other neurotransmitters have received less attention.

24. Answer: D
Sensory defensiveness is not considered a developmental disability.

25. Answer: D
Rocking slowly on a person's lap or in a rocker is a calming, not arousing, activity.

26. Answer: D
Having the child place his hands in wet oatmeal would be a good activity for a child if he has sensory defensiveness problems. Answers A, B, and C are all recommendations to increase hand strength.

27. Answer: D
You would not want to dress the patient yourself; as an OTA, you want to encourage independence. Answers A, B, and C are all suggestions to help the patient become more independent.

28. Answer: D
According to Mulley, answer D is correct because it carries less of a negative connotation than the term retirement. Answers B and C are terms for the same stage according to the author. Answer A is not an appropriate term for retirement.

29. Answer: C
Visual processing speed, ability to see well in dim light, and reading small print (near vision) all decline with age.

30. Answer: C
As an entry-level OTA, close supervision is required. General supervision is required for an intermediate-level OTA, and routine supervision is required for an advanced-level OTA.

31. Answer: B
The OT must select evaluation instruments, but the OTA may administer some of the evaluations. Answers A, C, and D are all roles of an OTA.

32. Answer: D
In the initial phases of the relationship, the most important role is that of listener. Answer A is not likely because giving advice often tells a person that the primary interest is in the content rather than the feelings being expressed. Answer B is not likely because it does not communicate to the patient that the message is being heard. Answer C is not likely because reassurance can limit further communication with the patient.

33. Answer: C
Although the patient's comfort is important, answers A, B, and D are all crucial reasons to keep a patient in proper body alignment.

34. Answer: A
An initial evaluation report does not include a treatment progress section because treatment of the patient has not yet begun at that point in time. Answers B, C, and D are all sections that should be included in the report.

35. Answer: B
Endurance is not generally a focus of treatment for a patient with Parkinson's disease. Answers A, C, and D are all important treatment goals for Parkinson's disease.

36. Answer: A
Generally, stroke does not seem to affect hearing, even in patients with aphasia. Answers B, C, and D are all common problems associated with a CVA.

37. Answer: D
The OTA will want to approach the child from the front (in his or her view) and apply firm pressure. All other answers are not likely because light touch should not be used, and the child should always be approached from the front.

38. Answer: C
After a THR, positions of instability are adduction, internal rotation, and flexion. Answers A, B, and D are unlikely.

39. Answer: C
Structuring the environment and cueing the patient will break down the activity, establish a routine, and help to increase independence during the activity. Answer A may be needed as the Alzheimer's becomes more severe. Answer B is unlikely because understanding written directions may be difficult for people with Alzheimer's dementia. Answer D is not likely because often times patients with Alzheimer's cannot initiate the activity.

40. Answer: B

Although perspiration, increased heart rate, and nausea may occur during a panic attack, extreme fear and sense of death are the major symptoms of a panic attack. Answer D is incorrect.

41. Answer: A

Increasing strength is not a priority treatment goal with the diagnosis of RA, while answers B, C, and D are all immediate areas to be addressed.

42. Answer: D

Mania is not a clinical feature of PTSD but is often seen instead in bipolar I disorder. Answers A, B, and C are all clinical features of PTSD.

43. Answer: D

The OTA must observe the child in the classroom to better understand how the child functions in his or her natural environment. Answers A, B, and C can be used to screen a child but are not as effective as observing the child functioning in the classroom.

44. Answer: B

The OTA would not necessarily be as concerned with the child's grade level directly but may use this information to support handwriting issues. Answers A, C, and D are important areas to look at when assessing handwriting.

45. Answer: D

The cause of schizophrenia is unknown. There are, however, theories supporting chemical imbalances, brain lesions, or environmental factors as the cause, but currently no scientific proof has been generated in the literature.

46. Answer: A

Claudia Allen developed the ACL, the RTI, and the ADM to determine what cognitive levels the client would be placed in (cognitive disabilities frame of reference). Mosey developed the group leveling system, placing people into groups from parallel to mature, numbering them 1 to 5. Lorna Jean King applied sensory integration theory to the treatment of psychiatric disorders. Gary Kielhofner developed the Model of Human Occupation.

47. Answer: C

The patient is instructed to not flex the hip greater than 90 degrees. A THR patient can put full weight on the nonsurgical side and is often allowed to use a toe-touch on the surgical side for balance. Although the patient should avoid internal rotation, he should not go to extremes of external rotation, but remain neutral.

48. Answer: A

In the early stages of the disease, emphasis is placed on strengthening exercises. Answer B is not likely because although talking and emotional support are parts of treatment and patient education, he is worried about fine motor performance. The patient is motivated to regain fine motor skills and strength, not equipment use. The shoulder and elbow are involved in gross motor function rather than fine motor.

49. Answer: D

It is typically difficult to interest a person with autism in new activities. Answers A, B, and C are all known characteristics of a person with autism.

50. Answer: C

The body righting on head reactions enables trunk movement to follow head movement; therefore, C is the best answer. By 7 months, the child is able to sit. In order to creep, the child needs to be able to support him- or herself, and the child should have the control to be able to stand by 10 months. In order to stand, the child has to learn all of the above first.

Section Five

1. Sensory loss, perceptual or cognitive dysfunction, and visual field deficits are all factors related to what disorder?
   A. Presbyopia
   B. Macular degeneration
   C. Unilateral neglect
   D. Hemianopsia

2. In general, tasks that are unstructured and creative tend to:
   A. Foster a sense of independence among lower-functioning persons
   B. Develop new coping mechanisms for lower-functioning individuals
   C. Increase the attention span of lower-functioning persons
   D. Make lower-functioning people feel inferior

3. The three subsystems identified by Kielhofner that interact to produce occupational acts are volition, habituation, and mind-brain-body performance. What subsystem is often, but not always, considered the starting point of any action?
   A. Mind-brain-body performance
   B. Habituation
   C. Communication interaction
   D. Volition

4. Which of the following is *not* an instrumental ADL?
   A. Communication
   B. Home management
   C. Safety management
   D. Nutrition

5. OTAs can be effective consultants in alternatives to restraints. All of the following would be alternatives to reduce restraints *except*:
   A. Replacing a belt or vest restraint with a reclined chair
   B. Personal alarm attached to the chair
   C. Wrap-around walker
   D. Directional signs placed in clear view of the patient

6. The OTA asks Mrs. Smith if she is able to toilet independently, and she responds that she is competent in this area. The OTA should:
   A. Accept the patient's statement
   B. Observe the patient to determine toilet independence
   C. Check with the aide and ask if she has observed the patient toileting
   D. Follow the doctor's admission note that the patient can transfer from bed to wheelchair independently

7. Mr. Ramos is an elderly man who is active in his group of friends. The "guys" love bowling on Friday nights. Mr. Ramos always wears his lucky shirt with the team logo and never fails to shine his bowling ball. What subsystem of the Model of Human Occupation influences Mr. Ramos' choice to regularly participate in the sport of bowling?

   A. Habituation

   B. Mind-brain-body

   C. Volition

   D. Personal causation

8. The occupational therapy team should only recommend discharge after:

   A. Re-evaluation

   B. Home evaluation

   C. Summary report

   D. Solution development

9. When an OTA is handed a referral by a doctor, the referral must be given to:

   A. A member of the treatment team

   B. The supervising OT

   C. The case management nurse

   D. The activity director

10. What two processes must take place before an individual treatment plan can be formulated?

    A. Screening and evaluation

    B. Short- and long-term goal development

    C. Problem and solution development

    D. Activity analysis and gradation

11. Bipolar disease is a combination of what two disorders?

    A. Depression and panic disorder

    B. Mania and panic disorder

    C. Panic disorder and dysthymia

    D. Depression and mania

12. Which statement *best* defines a "tip pinch"?

    A. Used to exert power on or with a small object

    B. Marked by significant wrist extension

    C. Used to obtain small items

    D. Used when strength of a grasp must be maintained to carry objects

13. A TBI patient that requires maximum assistance for new learning, follows simple directions consistently, and is now functional for common daily activities is at what RLA level?

    A. RLA IV confused-agitated

    B. RLA V confused-inappropriate, non-agitated

    C. RLA VI confused-appropriate

    D. RLA VII automatic-appropriate

14. In a warm-up session with a student who is seen for an instructional writing program, what activity should the OTA schedule *immediately* prior to the writing activity?
   A. In-hand manipulation activities, such as moving a 3/4" cube from palm to fingertips for stacking
   B. Visual perception activities, such as completing pencil and paper mazes that require staying within two lines
   C. Motor planning activities, such as cutting construction paper with scissors
   D. Postural preparation activities, such as wall push-ups

15. The four levels of supervision for occupational therapy practitioners include all of the following *except*:
   A. Minimal
   B. Close
   C. Routine
   D. Continuous

16. A patient exhibits akinesia from long-term use of a psychiatric medication. What should be done during her treatment sessions in order to compensate for this?
   A. Use gross motor activities and avoid resistance
   B. Select activities that allow the patient to stand up and do not prolong sitting
   C. Permit breaks in the activity and avoid activities with resistance
   D. Do not engage in fine motor activities and avoid power tools

17. What activity would *best* assist a child who has difficulty with supination of the forearm?
   A. Playing the card game "war" with the child's elbow in a fully flexed position throughout most of the activity
   B. Have the child toss a Nerf ball into a basket a few feet away. The elbow would be in extension for most of the activity
   C. Have the child take a wheelbarrow position and go through a small obstacle course with your assistance
   D. Have the child place various shaped blocks in a shape-sorter container

18. In wheelchair safety, what should be your primary precaution when transferring a patient out of the wheelchair?
   A. Look for obstacles that would prevent the patient from standing up
   B. Lock the brakes of the wheelchair
   C. Make sure there are no distractions
   D. Move the leg rest out to the side of the wheelchair

19. When working on hand skill development, what is the *first* intervention to perform?
   A. Have the child perform isolated finger movement activities using hand play songs
   B. In-hand manipulation activities with small toys
   C. Inhibit or facilitate tone as needed using specific techniques
   D. Position the child for stability to improve function during the activity

20. While performing a treatment group in a crowded room, you notice that a couple of members are having trouble hearing what is being said. The two members keep asking you to repeat the instructions by stating, "What were you talking about?" These members also had trouble conversing with the others and were constantly asking, "What did you say?" when another member addressed a question to them. In the end, these two members did not accomplish their goals. For the next group, what is the *best* method to help diminish this problem when performing activities?

    A. Check to make sure the patients have their hearing aids in

    B. Talk in a loud voice, so everyone hears you

    C. Go into a quiet area, such as a corner of a room

    D. Perform an activity that does not require much conversation

21. As an entry-level OTA, you see another OTA tell an aide to do a weight-bearing activity with a stroke patient. What should you do about this situation?

    A. Let it go. The supervising OT will see it and make sure that it will never happen again

    B. Do nothing. The aide may perform this activity because it is predictable

    C. Inform the OTA that an aide is not to perform any non-predictable activities

    D. During the aide's treatment session, go over to him and make sure he is performing the task correctly

22. What is the normal sequence in the development of grasp?

    A. Ulnar grasp to radial grasp to palmar grasp

    B. Radial grasp to ulnar grasp to palmar grasp

    C. Palmar grasp to ulnar grasp to radial grasp

    D. Ulnar grasp to palmar grasp to radial grasp

23. After a right CVA, a patient comes into your facility with her arm flexed in an involuntary reflex pattern. What is the correct name for this pattern?

    A. Spasticity

    B. Flaccid paralysis

    C. Synergy

    D. Paresis

24. A patient has a proximal interphalangeal (PIP) hyperextension and a distal interphalangeal (DIP) flexion in his fingers. What is this condition called?

    A. Boutonnière deformity

    B. Heberden's nodes

    C. Trigger finger

    D. Swan-neck deformity

25. You have noticed that one of the OTAs you are working with has just performed an unethical activity with a patient. Later that day you discussed with her the situation that had occurred. The next day you notice that the OTA does the same unethical activity. Which of the following would be the *next* step that you would take to deal with the situation?

    A. Ignore the situation for now and hope she learns on her own

    B. Report the situation to the OT supervisor and licensure board

    C. Discuss the situation with her one more time

    D. Recommend to the OT supervisor that she work with another patient

26. Your 70-year-old nursing home patient has difficulty concentrating during your treatment sessions. She admits she has difficulty sleeping, causing her to tire easily, and she cannot remain focused on her therapy. Although she would like to participate in the home's activities, she feels anxious in a group setting and prefers not to leave her room. What type of intervention would she *best* benefit from?

    A. Ask her medical doctor to prescribe a mild sedative to allow her to gain more rest in hopes that she will be more productive in her sessions

    B. Request a change to transfer your patient to a private room with no roommates

    C. Invite her to a small, one- to two-person group session that includes small arts and crafts activities, such as drawing, sewing, or bead work

    D. Reduce the workload of your sessions, and encourage her to be active by reading in her room

27. An OTA is providing OT services to a 3-year-old child with moderate spasticity secondary to CP. During the treatment session, the child has a momentary loss of awareness with no motor activity except eye rolling. Which of the following conditions should the OTA suspect?

    A. Mental retardation

    B. Anoxia

    C. Seizure

    D. Nystagmus

28. Symptoms such as a pounding headache, anxiety, perspiration, flushing of the skin, chills, nasal congestion, hypertension, and bradycardia would most likely be:

    A. Autonomic dysreflexia

    B. Orthostatic hypotension

    C. Brown-Séquard's syndrome

    D. Nystagmus

29. As the lens of the eye ages, it loses some of its elasticity. This condition is called presbyopia and is characterized by:

    A. Difficulty seeing at a distance

    B. Difficulty reading small print

    C. Loss of the central field of vision

    D. Blurred vision

30. Which of the following would *not* be an example of proprioceptive stimulation?

    A. Stretching exercises

    B. Lifting free weights

    C. Short-term memory games

    D. Resistance training

31. The onset of autism occurs at what age range?

    A. Prenatal to 2 months

    B. Birth up to the age of 30 months

    C. 3 to 5 years

    D. 5 to 8 years

32. Which of the following is the *first* step when providing treatment to improve hand and arm function of a 4-year-old girl with a brachial plexus injury?
    A. Inhibit tone
    B. Facilitate tone
    C. Position the child
    D. Provide PROM

33. What is the *best* bed position for a left-affected CVA patient to enable him to use the call bell during the night?
    A. Lying on the left side with pillows
    B. Lying on the right side with pillows
    C. Patient semireclined in bed
    D. Supine with extremities elevated

34. In the development of postural control for children, upon what basic assumption is NDT based?
    A. The decrease of abnormal postural tone to reduce hypertonicity in spastic and athetoid patients
    B. The facilitation of normal movement
    C. The use of righting and equilibrium reactions to improve functional skills
    D. All of the above

35. Which of the following abilities or capabilities does a patient with a C5 SCI share with a C6 SCI?
    A. May drive with one or more adaptations
    B. Can roll over or reach sitting position while in bed
    C. Is able to dress with little or no assistance
    D. Can perform skin inspections

36. An intermediate-level OTA who has just been hired at your facility proceeds to perform a treatment technique that she has never done before on a patient. When questioned, she sees nothing wrong with performing the treatment technique she saw in a book. What has the OTA *not* proven according to the OT guidelines?
    A. Honesty
    B. Confidentiality
    C. Competence
    D. Professional responsibility

37. As an entry-level OTA, who can you supervise at your facility?
    A. Aides, technicians, and volunteers
    B. Level I OT fieldwork students
    C. Other entry-level OTAs
    D. Level I and II OTA fieldwork students

38. All of the following are primary changes in the aging process *except*:
    A. Wrinkles
    B. Poor posture
    C. Sight changes
    D. Hearing changes

39. In what month of prenatal development does a fetus develop a grasp reflex?
    A. Month 3
    B. Month 4
    C. Month 6
    D. Month 8

40. After demonstrating competence, the OTA can perform the following assessments independently *except*:
    A. KELS
    B. BaFPE
    C. MEDLS
    D. ADL observation

41. What is the benefit of using standard assessments for ADLs?
    A. Admission and discharge scores can be used for outcome studies
    B. There is consistency between OTs and OTAs
    C. Validity and reliability scores improve the respect of occupational therapy with others
    D. All of the above

42. Mary is a 4-year-old girl who hates to be picked up and touched, even by her mother. She only eats puréed food and does not like the feeling of shirt tags on the back of her clothing. What would you suspect Mary has?
    A. Hyporesponsiveness
    B. Gravitational insecurity
    C. Sensory defensiveness
    D. Tactile defensiveness

43. Billy is a 45-year-old man diagnosed with cancer. He has a weak pelvic floor, which causes him to urinate on himself whenever he laughs or coughs. Billy is *most* likely suffering from what?
    A. Urge incontinence
    B. Overflow incontinence
    C. Stress incontinence
    D. Functional incontinence

Use the case study below to answer questions 44 to 46.

Mrs. Romano is a 43-year-old quilter who moved to the United States from Brazil 2 years ago. She moved here with her husband and her two children, ages 3 and 6. Mrs. Romano plays an active role in her community. She often volunteers for potluck suppers, arts and crafts, and other activities. She understands English quite well but can only speak a few common phrases. Mrs. Romano is left hand dominant and lives with her husband and two children on a top floor apartment in the city. One month ago, she was involved in a car accident and was injured. In the accident, Mrs. Romano suffered a fractured hip, a complete fracture in her left ulna, and some bruises. The doctor was able to put a cast on her left wrist, which is expected to heal quickly. Unfortunately, Mrs. Romano needed a THR. Mrs. Romano has been referred to OT for physical restoration. She is unable to perform in several ADLs.

44. Which of the following will Mrs. Romano *most* likely have difficulty with?
    A. Dressing and oral hygiene
    B. Toilet hygiene and eating
    C. Grooming and bathing
    D. All of the above

45. Due to Mrs. Romano's THR, the movement precautions are usually observed for how long?
    A. 2 to 4 weeks
    B. 6 to 12 weeks
    C. 8 to 10 weeks
    D. 10 to 14 weeks

46. Mrs. Romano has difficulty dressing herself. When provided with the correct assistive devices, she can dress with less difficulty. What is *least* effective for assisting a person with THR in dressing?
    A. Reacher
    B. Leg lifter
    C. Elastic shoelace
    D. Long handle shoehorn

47. What is the *least* effective use of an OTA's role in hospice?
    A. Explore the interests of the patient
    B. Educate on energy conservation
    C. Increase self-esteem
    D. Teach use of a wheelchair or walker

48. You are working with an aide in your facility. She is experienced and feels that she can handle more responsibility. When she suggests that she knows how to do a transfer because she has seen it done so many times, you tell her this is not allowed. Out of this list, what is another task that she cannot do?
    A. Work with patients in which the outcome is predictable
    B. Assist the OTA in doing an ADL assessment
    C. Setting up the area of therapy
    D. Work with the patient in an environment and situation that will be stable

49. With a patient initially being introduced to a wheelchair, what is *not* a correct safety element to teach?
    A. When pushing the patient down a ramp, the caregiver should tilt the wheelchair backward while descending
    B. During a transfer, the brakes should always be locked
    C. When pushing the patient up a ramp, the caregiver should have the patient assist
    D. Footplates should never be stood upon; when doing transfers, they should be in the up position

50. Which is not a complication after a CVA?
    A. DVT
    B. Subluxation
    C. Autonomic dysreflexia
    D. Seizures

Section Five Answers and Explanations

1. Answer: C
Unilateral neglect can be a combination of one or more factors, including perceptual or cognitive dysfunction, visual field deficits, and sensory loss. Answer A is not likely because presbyopia affects an individual's ability to see at near distances. Answer B is not likely because macular degeneration only affects the central vision. Answer D in not correct because hemianopsia is loss of visual field in the corresponding right and left half of each eye.

2. Answer: D
People who are cognitively low functioning need structure and predictability in their task performance. The unstructured, creative tasks tend to make these individuals feel worse because they are not able to accomplish a goal; thus, self-esteem may falter.

3. Answer: D
Volition is the correct answer because an individual must possess the desire, values, and interest before motivated to start any action. Mind-brain-body are the physical and mental skills that enable performance. Habituation is action that results from established patterns that repeat again and again. Answer C is not a good answer because communication interaction relates to skills of the mind-brain-body subsystem, which was developed by Kielhofner and his colleagues.

4. Answer: A
Communication is an ADL according to performance areas in the occupational performance domain of concern. Answers B, C, and D are listed as IADLs according to the occupational performance domain of concern.

5. Answer: A
Answer A is the most unacceptable method of restraint reduction. Answer B is a good form of restraint because it alerts the staff without preventing the elder from rising. Answer C uses the wrap-around walker to enable the elder to walk and be as independent as possible. Answer D implements directional signs, which enable the patient to find his or her way.

6. Answer: B
The OTA should never substitute her observations for the patient's word. Answers A, C, and D all describe observations or declarations made by others. It is always best to observe directly the actions of a patient before recording your findings as a caregiver.

7. Answer: C
It is volition that motivates individuals to participate in any activity. Answer A is not a good choice because habituation addresses internalized roles that cause an individual to act. Answer B would not apply because this subsystem is concerned with skills and rules and how to use them. Answer D is not likely because this is an individual's sense of his or her own competence and ability to be effective.

8. Answer: A
The re-evaluation process must always be implemented before the discharge process can take place. Answer B, C, and D are considered part of the discharge plan.

9. Answer: B
Answer B is the correct answer because it is the OTA's responsibility to give the supervising OT the referral as soon as the referral is received.

10. Answer: A
Screening and evaluation are the foundations for any implemented treatment plan. Answer B is not a likely answer because the short- and long-term goals must be established within the treatment plan. Answers C and D are also standard practices in the treatment plan.

11. Answer: D

Answer D is correct. This is the combination called bipolar disease. Answers A, B, and C may appear together in the diagnosis of a patient but are not the primary symptoms of bipolar disease.

12. Answer: C

Power grasp describes opposition of the thumb and index fingertip to obtain small objects. Answer A describes a lateral pinch. Answer B describes a spherical grasp. Answer D describes a hook grasp.

13. Answer: C

The person is only able to follow simple directions and has difficulty learning new things, which is characteristic of this RLA level. Answer A, RLA IV, is less likely. At this level the person cannot perform activities without maximum assistance and is unable to process information. RLA V is less likely because the person is still highly distracted and still requires assistance with activities. RLA VII is not likely because as confusion lessens, the person can follow more than simple directions and is capable of learning simple tasks.

14. Answer: D

Answers A, B, and C's activities may be part of the warm-up session; however, just prior to the handwriting session, postural preparations should be performed. Frequently, children with handwriting dysfunction experience poor proximal joint stability. Postural preparation activities encourage co-contraction through the neck, shoulder, elbows, and wrists.

15. Answer: D

Continuous supervision is for aides who need this type of supervision. Answers A, B, and C are levels of supervision for OT practitioners at various stages of experience.

16. Answer: C

Akinesia is the lack of physical movement. Permitting breaks and avoiding resistance are recommendations for adaptations and interventions associated with this side effect. Answer A includes adaptations and interventions associated with parkinsonism, a side effect characterized by muscular rigidity, tremors, drooling, shuffling gait, and mask-like face. Answer B includes adaptations and interventions associated with akathisia, a side effect characterized by restlessness and muscular tension. Answer D includes adaptations and interventions associated with dystonia, a side effect characterized by painful, sudden muscle spasm.

17. Answer: A

Supination is easiest to achieve when the elbow is fully flexed. Turning of cards requires movement of the forearm into supination. Supination is more difficult when the elbow is extended. Answers B and C are unlikely because the arm would be extended often in these activities. Answers C and D are unlikely because the activities require no supination of the forearm.

18. Answer: B

Locking the brakes is primary because it ensures that the chair will not move during the transfer, thereby reducing the risk of the patient falling. Answers A, C, and D are all important; however, they are not the primary safety precaution.

19. Answer: D

A secure base of support is important for optimal performance in any activity. Performance of activities listed in answers A, B, and C are automatically improved after proper positioning for stability.

20. Answer: C

Answer C is most likely because performing the group in a corner of a room can help diminish the sounds. Although answer A is possible, it is less likely because it does not address the noise in the room. Answer B is less likely because talking in a loud voice only makes it more confusing for the person while trying to hear you. Answer D is less likely because you want to promote conversation during an activity.

21. Answer: C
Weight-bearing is a non-predictable activity. Aides are only allowed to carry out treatment if the activity's outcome is predictable.

22. Answer: D
Answer D is the correct sequence of grasp development. Answers A, B, and C are incorrect sequences of grasp development.

23. Answer: C
The patient is presenting with a flexion synergy pattern of the upper affected extremity. A synergy is characterized by a group of muscles acting as a bound unit, resulting in an inability to perform isolated movements. Answer A refers to increased muscle tone. Answers B and D present as low tone and would not cause the upper extremity flexion. Additionally, flaccidity is usually the result of a peripheral nerve injury.

24. Answer: D
Swan-neck deformity is characterized by the position of the PIP joint in hyperextension and the DIP joint in flexion. Boutonnière deformity, which causes hyperextension of the DIP and extension of the PIP, is not possible because the extensor tendon slips below the axis of the PIP joint, causing it to become a flexed joint, which then hyperextends the DIP joint where they insert. Heberden's nodes are associated with OA and only affect the DIP joints. Trigger finger is incorrect because full extension of the PIP joint is prevented by restrictions of the FDS tendon.

25. Answer: B
According to the *Code of Ethics*, you should report the incident to the appropriate body, which includes supervisors, state agencies, NBCOT, and AOTA. Ignoring the situation will not solve the problem. If she has not corrected her behavior, she may continue to perform unethically. Answer D is less likely because she may perform unethically with another patient if the first problem is not dealt with.

26. Answer: C
Small group work engages the anxious patient with creative and repetitive activities (expressive therapies). Answers A, B, and D are incorrect because they do not recognize that she is suffering from anxiety and only encourage her fears.

27. Answer: C
Seizures are an associated problem of CP and are characterized by the description given. Answers A and D are associated with CP; however, they are not characterized by the symptoms given. Anoxia is a factor that may trigger a seizure; however, it is not a problem associated with CP and is therefore less likely.

28. Answer: A
Answer A is a condition caused by reflex action of the autonomic nervous system. Answer B is caused by lack of muscle tone in the abdomen, which leads to pooling of blood followed by hypotension. Answer C refers to motor paralysis and loss of proprioception by injury to only one side of the spinal cord. Answer D describes rapid involuntary movement of the eyes.

29. Answer: D
Presbyopia is associated with blurred vision. Answer A is associated with myopia. Answer B is associated with hyperopia. Answer C is associated with macular degeneration.

30. Answer: C
Answer C is incorrect because it is a cognitive activity. Answers A, B, and D are activities that stimulate the joint and muscle receptor.

31. Answer: B
Onset of autism can occur at birth or anytime up to 30 months of age.

32. Answer: C

Positioning is usually the first step in preparing a child for treatment of hand and arm function. Answers A, B, and D would be done after positioning.

33. Answer: A

The patient should lay on the affected side with the patient's back parallel to the edge of the bed. This position allows the use of the functional arm. Answer B is incorrect because the patient would be positioned on the unaffected arm, making the call bell difficult to reach. Answer C is incorrect because semi-reclined is not a typical sleeping position and is not beneficial for positioning of the affected limb. Answer D is incorrect because long periods of extreme flexion should be avoided in the affected limbs.

34. Answer: D

NDT is based on all of these characteristics.

35. Answer: A

Answer A is most likely, assuming that it is a complete injury. Answer B is incorrect because a person with a C5 SCI cannot perform this activity due to the lack of elbow extension, pronation, and all wrist and hand movements. Answers C and D are incorrect because a person with a C5 injury presents with total paralysis of trunk and lower extremities.

36. Answer: C

Competency, according to the guidelines, is developing new areas of skills and techniques and engaging in appropriate study and training. Answer A is less likely because the issue is being competent more than being honest. Answer B is not the issue for either OTA. Answer D is less likely because the problem at hand is the competency level, although professional responsibility consists of the occupational therapy practitioner having an obligation to maintain the standards of ethics.

37. Answer: A

Answer A is correct because the aides, technicians, and volunteers have less knowledge of the practice and need continuous supervision when working with patients.

38. Answer: B

Answer B is most likely because wrinkles, vision changes, and hearing problems are all primary changes in the aging process.

39. Answer: C

Grasp reflex develops in pre-natal month 6. In month 3, the fetus kicks and makes a fist. In month 4 of prebirth development, the fetus begins sucking, sleeping, and waking. In pre-natal month 8, the startle reflex is developing.

40. Answer: B

The KELS, MEDLS, and ADL observations are ADL assessments that the OTA can administer. Interpretation is done in collaboration with the supervising OT. The BaFPE is a functional, standardized assessment that requires OT credentials to administer.

41. Answer: D

Outcome measurement studies, practitioner consistency, and respect for the profession are all reasons to use published assessments.

42. Answer: D

Hyporesponsiveness may seek large quantities of intense stimulation when introduced to suspended equipment. Gravitational insecurity is a form of hyporesponsivity to vestibular sensations, which detect linear movement. Sensory defensiveness is an over-reaction to touch, movement, sounds, odors, and tastes.

43. Answer: C

Stress incontinence is when a person has a weak pelvic floor, which causes urination when laughing or coughing. OTAs can instruct clients with exercises to improve this condition. Urge incontinence is the inability to hold urine for a long period of time. Overflow incontinence is a constant dribble. Functional incontinence is when a person has impaired cognition, which causes him to urinate on himself.

44. Answer: D

Answer D is most likely because Mrs. Romano will have difficulty in all ADLs.

45. Answer: B

Typically, movement precautions are observed for 6 to 12 weeks, depending on doctor's orders and the speed of healing. Patients with problems, such as possible dislocation, will have longer precautions.

46. Answer: C

Most adults prefer to use slip-on shoes, such as loafers, rather than fuss with elastic shoelaces, which can be difficult to manage. The OTA should recommend shoes with safe bottoms that grip the ground without being too sticky or too slippery. Often the patient can buy these types of shoes before surgery. A reacher, leg lifter, and long handle shoehorn are easily accepted and assist with dressing.

47. Answer: D

Physical therapists are often available to teach patients how to use a wheelchair and walker if needed. An OTA can explore the patient's interests, educate on energy conservation, and increase self-esteem by helping the person arrange end-of-life meaningful activities.

48. Answer: B

Although an aide can provide helpful information on a patient's level of ADLs, the aide does not help in an evaluation. Answers A, C, and D are tasks that a competent aide can complete.

49. Answer: C

The patient should be told to keep his or her arms inside the wheelchair when someone else is pushing to avoid injury; therefore, C is the best answer. Answers A, B, and D are correct ways of maintaining wheelchair safety.

50. Answer: C

Autonomic dysreflexia is a safety complication with SCIs. Answers A, B, and D are all complications that a person may have after a CVA.

Section Six

1. Which of the following is true of documentation?
   A. Documentation is part of a legal document
   B. The OTA has ultimate responsibility for documentation
   C. Revisions to the record can be made after the fact
   D. Documentation can include review and criticism of another health care worker

2. The Health Care Financing Administration (HCFA) Common Procedures Coding System is used for reimbursement of Medicare and other services. What are these codes commonly called?
   A. Classification codes
   B. Reimbursement codes
   C. Billing codes
   D. *Practice Framework*

3. A person is considered independent when he or she requires what level of assistance?
   A. Caregiver provides hands-on assistance
   B. Caregiver provides hands-on assistance at times
   C. Caregiver provides no physical assistance but is allowed occasional verbal cueing
   D. Caregiver provides no assistance

4. Except for rotational movement of joints, joint movements occur on all of the following *except*?
   A. Sagittal
   B. Frontal
   C. Horizontal
   D. Axis

5. What activity is *best* for tactile input and gross motor planning for a 6-year-old boy?
   A. Lying on a bench, swimming in air
   B. Lying in a large cardboard box and rolling forward and backward inside the box
   C. Hanging from monkey bars
   D. Dancing freely to country music

6. What game will *best* assist inhibiting tonic neck reflex?
   A. Child on all fours, holding a paper "snowball" between the chin and shoulder
   B. Child on his or her back, making "snow angels" on the mat
   C. Child on all fours, holding a toy between the chin and chest
   D. Child playing with toy in a large cardboard box

7. Manual muscle testing (MMT) is limited by all of the following *except*?
   A. Muscle endurance
   B. Muscle coordination
   C. Muscle contraction
   D. Examiner's skill

8. To reduce the resistance to muscles during MMT, the OTA should:
   A. Position the person in the vertical plane
   B. Apply light resistance
   C. Eliminate gravity
   D. Evaluate functional ROM

9. To encourage a client to be more assertive in making her needs known, the OTA should:
   A. Teach assertiveness training
   B. Have the client practice using "I" statements
   C. Ask other people, such as family and caregivers, to ask her for her opinion
   D. Use probing questions to discover her feelings

10. The fulcrum of a goniometer is all of the following *except*?
    A. Free moving to allow for movement of the joint
    B. Tight enough to hold the measurement
    C. Also called the axis or rivet
    D. Attached to the moveable bar

11. A child in the custody of the state will be discharged from services on his 18th birthday. What is the treatment priority during his teen years?
    A. Complete evaluation and treatment of performance components
    B. Referral to appropriate adult services
    C. Independent living skills
    D. Self-esteem development and family education

12. What activity is the *best* choice for evaluating a patient's general and task behaviors?
    A. Baking cookies
    B. Reheating pizza
    C. Enjoying lunch with a peer
    D. Playing ping-pong

13. A client makes a collage that is bleak and sterile in affect. The OTA might expect the following:
    A. The person is hallucinating and has delusions
    B. The person is sad, lacks energy, and might be depressed
    C. The person is expressing anxiety over past events
    D. The person has a personality disorder

14. When an assessment has verbatim directions, what does this mean?
    A. The OTA can adjust or grade the directions to the client
    B. The OTA can use verbal or non-verbal cueing
    C. The OTA can answer questions during the assessment
    D. The OTA must state the directions exactly as written

15. Functional ROM is:
    A. Less than normal ROM
    B. Not appropriate for screenings
    C. Measured with a goniometer
    D. Evaluated during the interview with the client

16. Effective co-activation of the neck, trunk, shoulder, and pelvic areas assists in the development of normal muscle tone. Co-activation means:
    A. Stabilization
    B. Movement
    C. Tone
    D. Integration

17. Clonus is typically found in what situation?
    A. Hypotonicity
    B. Flaccidity
    C. Hypertonicity
    D. Deep tendon reflexes

18. The OTA has been administering a specific assessment for several years when a physician asks about the reliability of the assessment. The OTA states that she will have to check the manual because she does not remember this information off the top of her head. Back in the office she sees the reliability score in the manual. What is a good and realistic reliability score?
    A. $r = 1.0$
    B. $r = 0.8$
    C. $r = 0.6$
    D. $r = 0.4$

19. A person with positive supporting reflex (PSR) would have difficulty in:
    A. Putting on shoes
    B. Sucking from a straw
    C. Performing ADLs when head is turned to one side
    D. Releasing objects

20. When cleaning a spill of bodily fluids, the OTA should use gloves, paper towels, and a proper waste container plus:
    A. Bleach
    B. A mixture of 50% bleach, 50% water
    C. A mixture of 25% bleach, 75% water
    D. A mixture of 10% bleach, 90% water

21. An insulin reaction results from too much insulin or too little food. If the client is alert and conscious, what is the typical treatment?
    A. This is a medical emergency, call for assistance
    B. The patient usually takes some type of sugar, such as orange juice
    C. The nurse administers additional insulin as needed
    D. Nothing special; the problem will pass normally

22. An elderly man caring for his impaired wife with Alzheimer's disease has asked the OTA for ideas of things to do with his wife at home. He has accepted nursing aide care and referral to support programs but is looking to "do something" with his wife like they used to on family evenings together. Her functioning is reduced, and he is worried that she "just stares at the TV all day." The OTA suggests:

    A. Winding yarn, shelling beans, or stringing beads

    B. Baking cookies

    C. Making a fruit salad

    D. Housekeeping

23. Individuals with decreased self-awareness will likely have problems with:

    A. Motivation

    B. Problem solving and safety

    C. Perceptual and motor planning

    D. Speed of processing

24. A 75-year-old nursing home resident is participating in a sewing group but is being rude to her peers and the OTA. This resident has a long history of living in abusive situations and is currently taking psychiatric medications. What is the *best* response from the OTA?

    A. Have her leave the group and spend some quiet time sewing alone in the OT clinic

    B. Have her return to the unit

    C. Remind her that her behavior cannot be accepted and that she knows how painful it can be to be verbally abused

    D. Ignore the negative behaviors and reinforce any positive interactions

25. After 40 years at the same company, a 64-year-old man has begun making arrangements with his personnel office for mandatory retirement at age 65. He has found the process overwhelming, confusing, and agitating and has sought assistance from the local senior advocacy program where you work. After the social worker has clarified all the financial and legal issues, she has referred the client to OT. In the hall, the social worker tells you the client is "a wreck about retirement." After an initial interview to establish rapport, what is the *best* action?

    A. Leisure exploration

    B. Retraining for another job of interest

    C. General assessment of performance components and areas

    D. Depression and anxiety scales

26. What safety issue is considered an ADL?

    A. Fire safety awareness

    B. Wheelchair mobility

    C. Ability to use the 911 system

    D. Response to a carbon monoxide detector

27. What type of equipment is suggested for a person who cannot step over the side of a bathtub independently?

    A. Shower grab bars

    B. Transfer tub bench

    C. Extra long bath mat

    D. Bath equipment such as a long-handled sponge

28. What stage of diet progression requires the patient to be able to chew?
    A. Stage I
    B. Stage II
    C. Stage III
    D. All stages

29. All of the following foods are considered thin liquids *except*?
    A. Ice cream
    B. Milk
    C. Fruit juice
    D. Milk shake

30. What movement is the basis for all prehension patterns?
    A. Thumb opposition
    B. Thumb flexion
    C. Finger flexion
    D. Wrist flexion

31. All of the following allow the OTA to incorporate NDT techniques into ADLs for a person with hemiplegia *except*?
    A. Weight-bearing of involved UE
    B. Hand-over-hand bilateral tasks
    C. Use of lapboard for the affected extremity
    D. Clasped hands, interlocked fingers

32. During a task group for low functioning people with schizophrenia, a patient states that he can fly. When the other patients ignore him, he yells the statement out again. After asking the patient to refrain from yelling because it upsets the group members, what should the OTA do *next*?
    A. Confront the delusion, and tell the person that humans do not fly
    B. Reality orient the person X3
    C. Tell the person that you would like to hear more about this after group
    D. Ignore the outburst

33. After group, a young woman tells you, "I want to share something with you, but you can't tell anyone." The *best* response is:
    A. To agree so that rapport is built
    B. To agree so rapport is built, but break the agreement if it is something dangerous
    C. To say, "I do not keep secrets well"
    D. To say that all information is shared with the treatment team because we all work together

34. The use of a scooter board is effective in developing:
    A. Gross motor planning
    B. Vestibular input
    C. Integration of two sides
    D. All of the above

35. What game does *not* encourage bilateral integration?
    A. Wheelbarrow
    B. Bunny hop
    C. Hopscotch
    D. "Ice" skating on the floor

36. The art teacher is asking for suggestions for activities that can meet both her goals and the development of fine motor skills in her 2nd-graders. Which of the following would be *least* effective?
    A. Dot-to-dot drawing
    B. Yarn pictures
    C. Finger painting
    D. Clay

37. The maintenance of the facility's ADL kitchen has been assigned to the OTA. The OTA has training in infection control but will also need:
    A. To follow food service (restaurant/public health) rules
    B. Basic home management techniques
    C. Food management techniques
    D. All of the above

38. Professional development and socialization are directed by faculty and accreditation rules while a student is in OTA school. Once entry-level practice is achieved, professional development is directed by:
    A. National Board of Certification in Occupational Therapy (NBCOT)
    B. American Occupational Therapy Association (AOTA)
    C. State licensure laws
    D. The OTA

39. At what age can a child ride a tricycle, throw a ball without losing balance, and copy a circle?
    A. 2
    B. 3
    C. 4
    D. 5

40. What precaution is needed when using heat before an activity with a person with arthritis?
    A. State licensure laws
    B. Reimbursement issues
    C. Heat less than 20 minutes
    D. Doctor's orders

41. What adaptive equipment is *least* effective for a client with instability?
    A. Reacher
    B. Nonskid mats
    C. Suction brushes
    D. Grab bars

42. All of the following are benefits to using a stump sock with a prosthesis *except*:
    A. Absorbs perspiration
    B. Cosmetic appearance
    C. Protects from irritation
    D. Adjusts to volume change and aids fit

43. Mr. Horton, a large and generally fit man, has had Parkinson's disease for 1 year and is having increased difficulty with self-feeding. What weight is *best* for wrist weights to decrease hand tremors in this person with Parkinson's disease?
    A. ¼ pound
    B. ½ pound
    C. 1 pound
    D. 2 pounds

44. The geripsychiatric unit of a long-term facility has just hired an OTA to lead groups. The unit has been without OT services for several months due to hiring issues. The last practitioner ran a variety of groups and was well received. The staff reports that now clients just sit around all day. The OTA observes that most clients are sitting alone, watching TV, or pacing the hall; a few are playing cards. What group might be the *first* step in developing an OT program?
    A. Task or project group
    B. Social skills group
    C. Movement group
    D. Cognitive assessment group

45. All of the following statements about hemiwalkers are true *except*:
    A. A hemiwalker is used on the same side of the injury
    B. A hemiwalker provides greater support than a cane
    C. A hemiwalker is typically used when a person cannot manage a walker due to weakness
    D. The proper sequence is hemiwalker, weak leg, strong leg

46. What technique assists in facilitating the CNS in a child with behavioral issues?
    A. Brushing
    B. Joint compression
    C. Neutral warmth
    D. Reflex-inhibiting postures

47. All of the following are joint protection techniques *except*:
    A. Using a tight grip to avoid falls, injuries, or slips
    B. Maintaining proper position and posture
    C. Distributing load over two or more joints
    D. Alternating light and heavy tasks

48. For a female victim of abuse, what technique is *best* for expressing anger?
    A. Progressive relaxation
    B. Imagery
    C. Craft project such as tin punch or leather stamping
    D. Biofeedback

49. A confused women recovering from a head injury has been transferred to a rehabilitation program. On her first day, she used the public phone to call 911 and told police she was being held against her wishes. She has refused OT and PT services. She currently will not leave her room, stating, "No one is going to force me to go anywhere." What is the *best* first step to get her to leave her room and come to the OT clinic?

    A. Serve dessert in the day room

    B. Set up a behavior modification program

    C. Send her an invitation to visit OT

    D. Wait a few days for her to calm herself and try again

50. A 23-year-old male riding a motorcycle without a helmet was hit by a car and received numerous orthopedic injuries and a head injury. He is currently using a memory book but still asks repetitive questions such as, "Where am I again?" It is clear that his rehabilitation will be long-term, and he is expected to stay in the subacute rehab program for 6 to 9 months. He keeps asking the OTA to "get him a joint to smoke." What is the *best* response?

    A. Say, "That is not possible; I'll lose my job"

    B. Ignore the comment and redirect

    C. Remind the client that he is in a rehabilitation hospital

    D. Educate the client to the negative effects of marijuana and head injury

Section Six Answers and Explanations

1. Answer: A
Documentation is a legal document that can be used in court. The OT has ultimate responsibility for documentation, but the OTA can be called to court to explain treatment. Revisions to a record are allowed but only when noted and explained. Avoid criticizing another health care worker in a note because of legal issues.

2. Answer: A
Classification codes are the correct term, as part of the Physician's Current Procedural Terminology (CPT). These classification terms describe services by physicians and other health care workers.

3. Answer: C
Independence is no physical or verbal cueing. The other answers describe supervision or standby assistance.

4. Answer: D
Axis describes the pivot of movement. Sagittal, frontal, and horizontal planes are the most common.

5. Answer: B
The cardboard box provides both tactile input and gross motor movement. The other activities provide for gross motor issues but limit tactile input.

6. Answer: A
The child holding his chin to shoulder is best. The OTA should discourage the chin to the chest. The box play encourages the shoulders forward but limits movement. The snow angels are more appropriate for bilateral integration.

7. Answer: C
Measurement of muscle contraction is the purpose of MMT. Endurance and coordination cannot be measured by MMT, and the examiner's skill will limit the effectiveness of the measurement.

8. Answer: C
Eliminating gravity by positioning the person in a horizontal plane will allow evaluation of muscle contractions. The vertical plane is used for stronger muscles. Lighter resistance is not used in MMT. Functional ROM may provide information about muscle strength against gravity but is an evaluation of joint movement not muscle strength.

9. Answer: B
Having the client use "I" statements will give her skills and practice in making her needs known. Assertiveness training, although helpful, is general education on skills and concepts. Probing or asking others to probe keeps the client in a passive mode.

10. Answer: D
The fulcrum is attached to the stationary bar. All other answers are true of the fulcrum.

11. Answer: C
Unfortunately, many children in the custody of the state were placed in services because of abuse or neglect in their family. The dysfunctional family is not likely to be able to support the young adult on his 18th birthday. In the teen years, performance components, including self-worth, are important, but the priority is helping this young man be independent in the community without the supports that are typical for young men making it out on their own.

12. Answer: A
Evaluating general and task behavior, such as using the COTE, is best served with an activity involving three or more steps. This allows for evaluation of cognitive, motor, and perceptual skills, as well as social skills with the OTA. The pizza does not have three steps, lunch only addresses social skills, and ping-pong only addresses motor issues.

13. Answer: B

A person who is sad is more likely to do a collage that is bleak and empty. A person with schizophrenia is more likely to have a disorganized collage, while a person with anxiety will use pictures that represent their stressors and feelings. There are many different types of personality disorders, resulting in many different types of collages.

14. Answer: D

The OTA must give the directions exactly as written and cannot give cues, answer questions, or adjust the evaluation unless the directions say so.

15. Answer: A

Functional ROM is less than normal but is is needed for typical ADLs, such as eating or grooming. Functional ROM is evaluated by watching a client move in a variety of directions and does not use a goniometer or interview. The OTA observes the movement.

16. Answer: A

Co-activation refers to stabilization. Stabilization is affected by reflexes and positioning.

17. Answer: C

Hypotonicity and flaccidity are the same. Hypertonicity or spasticity is characterized by hyper deep tendon reflexes and clonus. Clonus is quick and repetitive contractions of muscles.

18. Answer: B

A correlation of one ($r = 1.0$) would be considered perfect, meaning that the test has perfect reliability. Because this would be difficult to produce unless in perfect laboratory conditions, a reliability of 0.8 is very good and realistic. Any assessment with a reliability of 0.6 or higher is worth investigating for your specific population.

19. Answer: A

Putting on shoes would be difficult because the leg would be in extension. Sucking from a straw is from a suck reflex, ADLs with head turned is ATNR, and releasing is from palmar grasp reflex.

20. Answer: D

Spills of bodily fluids must be cleaned using bleach 1:10. In addition, gloves, paper towels, and an infectious waste container should be used.

21. Answer: B

A little sugar will likely stabilize the situation. The person should monitor the situation with blood sugar tests and stop physical activity until he or she feels better.

22. Answer: A

Winding yarn, stringing large beads, shelling nuts or beans, and sorting are repetitive activities that do not require much caregiver supervision. The other activities, although possible, require more supervision because of safety issues.

23. Answer: B

Self-awareness is needed to recognize problems, solve problems, and avoid safety issues. The other issues may be present, but without self-awareness a person is likely to put him- or herself in dangerous situations.

24. Answer: C

Remind the patient that you cannot allow her to be rude and abusive toward others in group. Reward her for positive interactions.

25. Answer: A

The client has had a structured life at the same facility for 40 years. His social situation is likely tied to his work as well. Although depression, anxiety, another job, or performance components might be an issue, he is likely upset about what he is going to do with his time without the meaningful activity of work. Explore leisure first to see what time-management skills he currently has.

26. Answer: B

Wheelchair mobility is considered an ADL, while the others are IADLs.

27. Answer: B

Grab bars, tub mat, and bath equipment might be helpful, but the transfer tub bench will allow the person to get over the side of the tub easily.

28. Answer: C

Stage I is puréed and stage II is mechanical soft foods that stay together in a bolus. Stage III requires chewing.

29. Answer: D

A milk shake is considered a semi-thick liquid, as are yogurt, nectars, and tomato juice. Thin liquids are water, coffee, fruit juice, milk, gelatin, ice cream, and sherbet.

30. Answer: A

Thumb opposition is the foundation of all prehension patterns. Finger flexion is required in most grasps but to a varying degree.

31. Answer: C

The lapboard is effective positioning to prevent shoulder problems during rest. The other techniques should be used during ADL activities using the NDT approach.

32. Answer: C

Confrontation, ignoring, or reality orientation does not work with a person who is actively delusional. The best response to a delusional statement is not reinforcing of the idea but rapport building, "That's very interesting. Tell me more about that."

33. Answer: D

Although rapport is important, the client may be setting the practitioner up with important information that must be shared. Probing questions and reassurance that the information will stay within the team should reassure the client, develop rapport, and address safety.

34. Answer: D

A scooter board can be effective in all of these areas depending on the specific task. Sitting on the board and being pulled by the OTA will be vestibular, while lying on the board and crawling is gross motor and bilateral integration.

35. Answer: C

"Ice" skating in socks on a gym floor, wheelbarrow, and bunny hop all require movement of both sides of the body, while hopscotch requires co-constriction of one side.

36. Answer: A

Although dot-to-dot drawings are an excellent fine motor activity, this activity would not meet the artistic goals of an art curriculum because it is a cognitive activity.

37. Answer: D

In addition to infection control, the OTA will need to follow several other agencies' rules on food preparation, including the local town's public health rules. In general, food needs to be dated and regularly checked, the area of preparation kept cleaned, and safety issues must be addressed.

38. Answer: D

Once practicing, OTAs are responsible for directing their own professional development and socialization. Requirements from outside agencies, including the facility at which the OTA works, may impact the choices of the OTA. It is the OTA's ultimate responsibility to stay current in practice.

39. Answer: B

A 2-year-old can run well and has an overhand grasp of crayons. A 4-year-old can manipulate a wagon, throw a ball overhand, and draw crude human figures. A 5-year-old can use skates, bounce large balls, and hop.

40. Answer: C

Heat must be kept at 20 minutes or less to reduce the chance of inflammation or edema from the heat. When edema is present, ice may provide pain relief. All the other answers are administrative issues related to the use of physical agent modalities and apply to the use of heat.

41. Answer: A

A reacher is typically used for decreased ROM and might be dangerous to a person with instability, in case of a fall. Non-skid mats, suction tools, handrails, and grab bars are effective for instability.

42. Answer: B

Similar to the same reasons people wear socks with shoes, stump socks of wool, cotton, or man-made fabrics absorb perspiration, protect from direct contact, adjust to limb changes, and aid in fit. However, stump socks are different from traditional socks in that they do not have a cosmetic purpose.

43. Answer: C

Begin with 1-pound weights and adjust from there.

44. Answer: C

Although all of these groups might be appropriate for this unit, the movement group is the best place to start because it is an alerting activity that will set the foundation for socializing and task making. A cognitive assessment, such as the ACL, will likely confirm information that is already known, since this is a long-term unit for older adults with psychiatric issues.

45. Answer: A

A hemiwalker is used opposite the injury. All the other statements are true.

46. Answer: A

Techniques to facilitate the CNS include brushing, icing, tapping, quick stretching, postural change, sensory stimulation, and vibration. Techniques to inhibit the CNS include neutral warmth, joint compression less than the person's body weight, reflex-inhibiting postures, slow rocking, slow rolling, slow stroking, and weight-bearing.

47. Answer: A

Avoid a tight grasp to protect hand joints. All other answers are joint protection techniques, including using legs to lift, avoiding the same position, taking rests, stopping when fatigued, reducing effort, and avoiding pressure on hands.

48. Answer: C

Activities that allow physical output of anger include many crafts, such as tin punch or leather stamping. The other answers are all relaxation techniques that would also be helpful in conjunction with the physical expression of her anger. Additional relaxation techniques include visualization, meditation, self-hypnosis, shoulder shrugs, and muscle tightening/releasing.

49. Answer: C

She has stated she does not want to be forced, so an invitation may be all she needs to feel control. A behavior modification program is too extreme to start with, and the client cannot miss several days of treatment due to reimbursement issues. The dessert may or may not be motivating, but is not the best choice with which to start.

50. Answer: B

At this stage of recovery, any attempt to educate would be frustrating to the client. It is best to redirect his attention and ignore the comment.

Chapter Six

Domain-Style Study Questions and Answers

Section One

1. A school system with a team approach to managing feeding and eating issues of students is interested in adding occupational therapy. What is the *first* priority for the new OTA team member?

   A. Proper positioning and safety issues regarding eating

   B. Providing interventions to increase developmental self-feeding

   C. Providing oral-motor interventions

   D. Assessing oral-motor issues

2. In evaluating a senior citizen's ability to keep a driver's license, the OTA is *first* concerned with:

   A. Visual skills

   B. Cognitive functioning

   C. Physical functioning

   D. Brake-reaction time

3. What position allows for gravity-assisted movement for play in a toddler with developmental issues?

   A. Supine

   B. Prone

   C. Side-lying

   D. Sitting

4. The nursing department in a skilled nursing and rehabilitation facility is asking the OT and OTA to assist with residents' hand care in the long-term program. These residents are not eligible for reimbursed OT services and have little rehabilitation potential, but the nurses are reporting that tight hands make bathing difficult. What should the OTA do?

   A. Recommend the nurses keep rolled up washcloths in the residents' hands

   B. Make or buy hand cones for all the residents

   C. Evaluate each resident's hands and recommend needed equipment without reimbursement

   D. Make verbal suggestions to the nursing department because the residents are not eligible for services

5. A company is considering hiring an OT and OTA team to consult with the employees about reducing musculoskeletal disorders and work absences. All of the following could be used to promote the use of OT at the work site *except*:

   A. The services could be billed under the medical insurance

   B. Reduced workers' compensation costs to the employer

   C. Respond to an Occupational Safety and Health Administration (OSHA) citation

   D. Respond to OSHA-proposed ergonomic standards

6. An individual who uses a power wheelchair and has severe contractures is developing pressure sores despite earlier low-technology interventions. The doctor has asked occupational therapy for an opinion on a tilt or recline system to relieve the pressure. What is likely the *most* effective?

   A. Tilt

   B. Recline

   C. Whichever would allow the client to transfer easiest

   D. Either one—consider cost and mobility first

7. An assisted-living facility has expressed some interest in finding out more about occupational therapy. Currently, an OTA from the local visiting nurse agency visits one of the residents for home therapy after a stroke. All of the following services are appropriate *except*:

   A. Consulting with residents through home evaluations on ways to reduce falls

   B. Consulting with administration on developing a social-emotional system that involves all residents

   C. Provide direct OT services billing through Medicare or Medicaid

   D. Educate family or home health aides on ways to better facilitate independence

8. The OTA working for a large school system has been assigned the additional responsibility of being the ADA consultant for the employees with disabilities. What is the *first* step in managing this task?

   A. Subscribe and read journals related to the ADA, workplace issues, and laws

   B. Call local human resources personnel and ask for copies of policies they use

   C. Attend training or conferences on the ADA advocacy

   D. Obtain and read the ADA and administrative guidelines from the Equal Employment Opportunity Commission

9. An OTA is working with an elderly man with peripheral visual field loss. As part of a grant from a local service club, the client is picked up at his home and transported to the outpatient clinic where the OTA works. The client has reported satisfaction with his treatment, and the OTA has arranged a home visit to evaluate the client's integration of learning to his context. During the home visit, his daughter reports how frustrated she is with her father knocking over cups of water during dinner when he reaches for other items. What should the OTA do to address this issue?

   A. Have the client switch to a sports bottle-type cup for water

   B. Teach the client to visually scan in an organized manner to avoid overlooking items on the table

   C. Have the daughter switch to a tablecloth that contrasts with the cup so the client will see it better

   D. Ask the eye doctor to address the issue during his next visit

10. A one-handed high school freshman athlete is at risk of losing his athletic status because of low grades. His teachers report that the major issue is not his cognitive understanding but his unreadable and messy work. The OTA reviews his record to see that he has been offered keyboarding techniques but prefers hand-writing because of speed. The student says that his athletic status is most important to him and does not understand why the teachers are "picking on" his handwriting. The student is willing to reconsider key-boarding issues to meet his goal. What is *most* important in successful one-handed keyboarding?

   A. Training

   B. Positioning

   C. Adapted keyboard

   D. Data-entry skills

11. A former client and his family have called your outpatient facility and reported that, because of their sat-isfaction with services rendered when they were in rehabilitation, they would like to pay for consulting services as they get ready to build a new house. The client would like to have the new house built with environmental controls and electronic aids to improve his management of ADLs. The licensure laws in this state allow for services to be rendered without doctor's orders, and the facility is interested in exploring new non-medical services. The architect needs to know what type of input the electronic devices will use. The client has UE movement and reports his most important goal is socializing. What inputs might be eval-uated *first*?

   A. Switch

   B. Voice

   C. Serial, computer

   D. Combination

12. A parent reports frustration with the attempt to encourage her child to stand. She adds that the child cries when standing and gets things done faster if allowed to crawl. The parent knows standing is important to walking but cannot handle the crying. The OTA recommends play activities during standing. What play activity during standing is *not* recommended?

   A. Singing and rocking side to side or front to back

   B. Bright socks and bells on the ankles

   C. Reaching for toys slightly out of reach

   D. Standing in front of a mirror

13. Children with ADHD may also have learning disabilities. The OT will do further evaluations, but what should the OTA observe for?

   A. Occupational performance

   B. ADLs

   C. Handwriting

   D. Memory

14. A client you are seeing for hand rehabilitation mentions that he also has gout and that it is flaring up because of all the picnics he went to over the long 4th of July weekend. He adds that his doctor did not give him any new medication because of the NSAIDs he is taking for his hand. He asks the OTA for rec-ommendations. The OTA recommends all of the following *except*:

   A. Reduce alcohol ingestion

   B. Consider a weight reduction program

   C. Restrict fluid intake to reduce swelling

   D. Keep the doctor updated on all other medications he is taking

15. A toddler with failure to thrive is referred for home evaluation and treatment for developmental issues. The toddler is below the fifth percentile for weight for her age. Her mother reports every meal is a battle. The OTA recommends all of the following *except*:

    A. Allow snacking and juice consumption throughout the day

    B. Incorporate play and playful interactions into meals

    C. Consider the child's emotional needs

    D. Consider age-appropriate portions of foods

16. A baby lying in supine is developing midline control, moving arms against gravity, and body awareness of the lower extremities. How can the parents facilitate gravity-resisted play?

    A. Put bracelets or rattles on the baby's ankles

    B. Have the parents make faces and sounds to attract the baby's interest

    C. Use a mirror to encourage the baby to lift his or her head

    D. Hold toys at different positions

17. An OTA has been asked for recommendations to help a third-grader stay in his classroom seat, as he usually wiggles around until standing and disrupts others. The student was getting services from special education, and his parents had him enrolled in a sensory integration program after school. What recommendation could result in improved focus on tasks?

    A. Replace the static classroom chair with an inflatable ball

    B. Evaluate for motor movement issues

    C. Replace the classroom chair with a firm chair with side arms

    D. Use a lap tray on a soft chair to keep the student focused

18. Changes in Medicare funding and insurance reimbursement have lead to changes in the traditional roles of occupational therapy practitioners. The *most* effective way to advocate for legislation that supports the profession is forming a collaboration with:

    A. Lawyers

    B. Medical doctors

    C. Other rehabilitation specialists, such as physical therapists

    D. Lobbyists

19. What type of visual supports are *most* effective for children with autism in the early stages of reading skills?

    A. Cue cards with objects and words

    B. Calendars and mini-calendars

    C. Checklists

    D. Semantic maps

20. A mother complains that her 11-year-old son "can't find his way out of the bathroom" and is worried he will become hopelessly lost when he goes to a new middle school next academic year. The OT evaluates the student for directional dysfunction and agrees with the mother that there is a problem. The OTA knows that rules at the middle school are tight to provide structure for the preteens, and lateness to class is not tolerated. The student is adamant that no one is to know he has a problem. His mother is supportive of this decision because she understands the peer pressure in middle school. The family has agreed to follow the OTA's recommendations and practice over the summer. The OTA has graded a list of activities that increases the level of directional skill. What is the *highest* level of directional skill?

    A. Body awareness

    B. Self as a reference point

    C. Environment as a reference point

    D. Others as a reference point

21. An OT and OTA team has been asked to consult with the family of a 69-year-old woman recovering from a left CVA. The woman is medically stable and will be leaving the acute care hospital for a 1-week rehabilitation stay in a local nursing facility. The family's priority is home care rehabilitation as soon as possible. The occupational therapy practitioners must consider assessment of all of the following *except*:

    A. Environment

    B. Social support

    C. Financial support

    D. Medical status at admission

22. The OT clinic must have available material safety data sheets (MSDS) on all of the following *except*:

    A. White-Out

    B. Theraputty

    C. Soaps

    D. Personal items

23. Often OTAs and OTs work together on the treatment of a particular client. What is the *best* way to document supervision of the treatment and OTA by the OT?

    A. The OT cosigns the treatment notes in the medical record

    B. The OT keeps a supervision logbook when discussing treatment with the OTA

    C. No special documentation is needed because billing is the same for OTAs and OTs

    D. A third party, such as the OT supervisor, documents the collaboration

24. During a preschool screening, the OTA observes abnormal hand movements such as hand wringing or hand washing, and the mother reports a loss of hand skill development. What diagnosis might be present?

    A. Childhood disintegrative disorder

    B. Childhood schizophrenia

    C. Autism

    D. Rett syndrome

25. What are the signs of SI dysfunction?

    A. Over-sensitivity to sound, movement, touch, or visual input

    B. Impulsivity, lack of self-control, distraction

    C. Poor self-concept, social problems

    D. All of the above

26. All of the following are contraindications for aquatic therapy *except*:
    A. Open wound
    B. Decreased cardiovascular endurance
    C. Incontinence
    D. Severe cardiovascular disease

27. The *best* activity to observe motor synthesis is:
    A. Playing hopscotch
    B. Guessing an object's name without looking at it
    C. Constructing a three-dimensional box out of paper
    D. Copying a two-dimensional block design

28. All of the following activities are suited to increase spatial relationship awareness *except*:
    A. Making a tall tower of blocks
    B. Doing arithmetic problems
    C. Drawing hands on a clock
    D. Drawing a designated object from memory

29. The *best* movement activity for persons with schizophrenia is:
    A. A routine exercise program
    B. Country line dancing
    C. Spontaneous movement to music
    D. Tap dancing

30. At what age can a child maintain head control when supported in sitting?
    A. 1 month
    B. 2 months
    C. 4 months
    D. 5 months

31. A child of 2 to 3 years old who grabs a chunky crayon with his fingers while his wrist is pronated is show-ing what type of grasp?
    A. Mature dynamic tripod
    B. Less mature static tripod
    C. Immature pronated grasp
    D. Power grasp

32. A group of parents have asked the OTA to prepare a short in-service on reflexes for the birth to 3-years-old program. All of the following are spinal cord level reflexes *except*:
    A. Rooting and sucking
    B. Flexor withdrawal and placing
    C. Stepping and gallant
    D. ATNR and STNR

33. A parent with a child who is newly diagnosed with CP wants the OTA to explain why her child looks so much different from the other children in the clinic. She understands that there are different classifications of CP and wants to know which one is "more common?"

    A. Spasticity

    B. Athetoid

    C. Flaccid/atonia

    D. Mixed

34. A Sunday school teacher has commented that she has several children that "don't act normal" in class. One parent has asked the OTA to educate all the teachers about PDD. All of the following are classified as PDD and should be included *except*:

    A. Autism

    B. Asperger's syndrome

    C. Rett syndrome

    D. Childhood schizophrenia

35. A child in a full inclusion classroom requires staff and parent education to succeed. The role of the occupational therapy practitioner includes all of the following *except*:

    A. Educate the teacher on body mechanics so the teacher does not hurt her back when moving the child

    B. Educate the parents on techniques to maintain performance in the classroom

    C. Advise the parents on medical procedures that can enhance classroom performance

    D. Educate the teacher's aid to optimum classroom positioning and seating for the child

36. A 17-year-old young man with autism has been successful in all his OT treatments except shaving. His female classroom teacher reports some peers are teasing him about his "5 o'clock shadow." The teenager lives at home with his single mother and two younger sisters. The mother is frustrated because she has to nag the teen to get him to shave in the morning. As the school-based consulting OTA, what is the *best* option for treatment?

    A. Have the teen wait to shave until he gets to school and then have his teacher supervise

    B. Allow the teen's beard to grow in and not shave at all

    C. Start a shaving group with all the young men in the teen's classroom

    D. Arrange a male teen volunteer to role model shaving with the young man

37. Sensory integration development continues throughout life, especially in active adults, but is generally complete by what age?

    A. 1 to 3 years of age

    B. 4 to 5 years of age

    C. 8 to 10 years of age

    D. 14 to 18 years of age

38. A person with a SCI who complains of dizziness and feels faint may be experiencing:

    A. Autonomic dysreflexia

    B. Pulmonary emboli

    C. Orthostatic hypotension

    D. Abdominal distention

39. In a pediatric population, what type of equipment is *most* effective for vestibular treatment?
    A. Suspended equipment
    B. ADL equipment
    C. Computer equipment
    D. Pen and paper tasks in a classroom

40. A blind or visually impaired person may have some sight. All of the following can assist the individual in his or her home environment *except*:
    A. Contrasting scatter rugs by the doors
    B. A dark placemat or cup on a light surface
    C. Stair risers painted in a contrasting color
    D. White tape to mark a dark object

41. When an elderly person has recently lost all vision, all of the following are helpful *except*:
    A. Textured surfaces to indicate the top and bottom of stairs
    B. Safety pins in different arrangements to mark clothes
    C. Textured doorknobs to mark exits
    D. Labels or signs in braille

42. As part of managed health care, cross training is used. This involves:
    A. OTAs co-treating the patient with a physical therapy assistant
    B. Many disciplines being able to meet the client's basic needs
    C. OTAs continuing their education to avoid being laid off
    D. OTAs being physically fit so they can work at maximum efficiency

43. A critical path is:
    A. A planned treatment schedule based on effective treatment approaches
    B. An environmental simulation that has different textures
    C. A warning that the patient may have an infectious disease
    D. Important documentation that is found in the front of the medical record

44. When should discharge plans begin?
    A. At admission
    B. Once the patient is out of the critical care unit
    C. When rehabilitation begins
    D. At least 1 week before the patient is ready for discharge

45. When a patient is frightened to transfer out of bed and into a wheelchair, the OTA should do all of the following *except*:
    A. Use a firm touch and hurried motions to make the transfer as quick as possible
    B. Tell the patient what you intend to do and how you will do it
    C. Answer "I can't" with "Yes you can, and I will help you"
    D. Instruct one step at a time

46. The best way to clean a wheelchair after it has been exposed to rain or snow is:
    A. Hose it down with clean water
    B. Let it air dry
    C. Use a light oil on the cross-brace center pin
    D. Wipe it dry with a cloth using a metal cleaner if needed

47. A person with Alzheimer's disease who is unable to manage bathing but is still able to choose the proper clothing for the season might indicate a differential diagnosis of:
    A. Arthritis
    B. Schizophrenia
    C. Myocardial infarction
    D. Multiple sclerosis

48. Signs of extra-pyramidal syndrome (EPS) include all of the following *except*:
    A. Lip puckering or smacking
    B. Inability to sustain tongue movement
    C. Frowning, blinking, smiling, or grimacing
    D. Arms rapidly moving without objective or slow athetoid movements

49. When teaching elderly clients about their medication routine, keep information short and to the point, be concrete about the time the medication should be taken, provide written directions at the end of the session, and:
    A. Use the words "drugs" or "pills" instead of the word "medicine"
    B. Ask the client to repeat the information back to you
    C. Use technical words as well as common language
    D. Change all bottles to easy-open caps

50. Which of the following alternatives to restraints for the confused elderly is *not* effective?
    A. Structured, predictable routine
    B. Several activities to choose from
    C. Validate feelings; if the resident is looking for his or her mother, attend to the feelings behind it
    D. Place names and pictures on the door

Section One Answers and Explanations

1. Answer: A

Safety is always first, and positioning aids in feeding. All the other answers are appropriate for the OTA to address, but safety is first.

2. Answer: B

All of the skills are important in driving, but cognitive skills can impact the other skills and affect the person's ability to make sound driving judgments.

3. Answer: C

Side-lying brings the child's arms and legs to midline and provides gravity assistance to movement for play. The child can see the hands and begin to coordinate movements. Pillows and rolled-up towels can support the position. The other positions require more resistance to gravity and may also be appropriate for addressing developmental issues.

4. Answer: C

If the occupational therapy practitioners are employed by the facility, services can be provided without reimbursement issues. If the OT staff is employed by a contracted agency, the facility likely has an arrangement that allows long-term residents to have access to services. The OT practitioners have an ethical responsibility to assure everyone has access to services. From a treatment perspective, answer A is rarely an acceptable plan. Soft washcloths only encourage flexion, making the problem worse. Hand cones or commercially available equipment that is shaped like a carrot is more appropriate. Nursing often uses washcloths and should be educated that this will make the hand tightness worse. The exception would include extremely fragile residents, whose quality of life is more important.

5. Answer: A

A company cannot bill its own ergonomics consultants under its own medical insurance. The company would have to pay for these services in some other way but would likely see reductions in medical and workers' compensation costs as employees reduced work-related injuries.

6. Answer: A

Tilt and recline wheelchairs are used for a variety of issues, including pressure relief, head and neck control, sleep, improved functional access, and regulating blood pressure. A tilt system does not change the angles of the body as does a recline system. The tilt is more appropriate for contractures that will not allow for changing body angles. Tilt and recline systems do add costs and weight to power chairs, and this needs to be considered as well.

7. Answer: C

Assisted-living centers promote independence. Although a person may be eligible for direct OT services through a third-party payer, the focus in assisted living is prevention.

8. Answer: D

All of the answers are good ways to become educated about the ADA; however, the OTA should first obtain the law and guidelines.

9. Answer: B

Adapted equipment is not considered until other issues are addressed. The issue is not just spilling water but overlooking items when looking for a different item. Changing the cup or tablecloth may be appropriate if the family does not mind the change, but many families have rituals at dinner, and a sports bottle or contrasting tablecloth might not fit their context. The eye doctor might be appropriate if other issues are involved but not necessarily appropriate if cognitive training addresses the problem.

10. Answer: B

Positioning includes the user's relationship of body to the keyboard, hand placement, size and range of motion of the hand, size of fingers, and the relationship to the size of keys. Training and keyboarding are addressed after position. In this specific class, the benefits in keyboarding will likely show immediate results in quality of academic work, allowing the student to maintain athletic status. The correct positioning will be less intrusive and likely not resisted by the teen. Positioning also reduces secondary disabilities like carpal tunnel syndrome, which could affect the athlete.

11. Answer: C

Computer electronic aids to daily living would be a logical first step because of the ability to increase socialization through chat rooms and email. Computers also provide the most variety for use over switches, which are on/off, or voice, which is limited to vocal commands. Switches and voice may also be used in selected areas of the house for specific needs, but computers allow greater socialization.

12. Answer: B

Bright socks or toys on the feet will encourage the child to look down and make balance less successful. The other play activities encourage correct position and balance, which are the needed skills for walking.

13. Answer: D

Deficits caused by a learning disability affect short-term memory, which may be used for spelling and reading. Memory may then heighten the ADHD symptoms. The other areas may be appropriate assessment for a student, but memory must be addressed first.

14. Answer: C

Gout is a condition of hyperuricemia, typically affecting the great toe but not limited to this joint. Acute swelling, pain, and hot joints result. Alcohol ingestion (especially beer), obesity, and low urine volume exacerbate gout. Some medications also affect the condition, so the client should also inform the doctor of other medications he is taking.

15. Answer: A

Snacking and juice throughout the day will mean the child is not hungry at mealtime. Picky eaters, especially toddlers, have special issues. First, many toddlers are picky eaters, and this passes with time. Toddlers are experimenting with the word "no" and often try this during meals. The child must trust the feeder, and other emotional needs must be met. The OT can model positive feeding behaviors if needed. Age-appropriate portions are often one-third to one-fourth an adult portion. Play during feeding can reduce stress and increase trust.

16. Answer: C

Using a mirror to encourage a baby to lift her head is most appropriate for prone position. The other activities encourage reach.

17. Answer: A

The ball allows for increased sensory input, so the student can stay focused on the task at his desk. The other chairs are restrictive and would not change the problem. There is no indication that there is a motor issue.

18. Answer: D

Collaboration with other people for the common good is beneficial. However, lobbyists are trained professionals that have the ear of senators and congress people who make changes in laws. A primary function of AOTA (and where member dues are used) is to advocate for the profession at the national and state legislative levels.

19. Answer: A

Cue cards with pictures and words help the student develop reading skills while also acting as visual reminders and reinforcing social skills. Cue cards without pictures are also helpful once the student begins reading. Calendars and semantic maps provide additional ways of organizing information once basic concepts are mastered.

20. Answer: D

Body awareness, self, environment, and others as reference is the development of directional skills. This student likely has body awareness and self as reference (intrapersonal space) mastered but needs to develop skills in extrapersonal space. Environment reference sees the body in relationship to objects in space. Others as a reference point understands that every person has a different perspective of direction than the child's perspective.

21. Answer: D

The OT team knows that she is medically stable before transfer to rehabilitation. Although an assessment of her functioning in the acute setting may be interesting, it likely will be of little assistance to her functioning after rehabilitation. Environmental changes require social support and, depending on the resources of the client, may include financial issues.

22. Answer: D

MSDS are required to protect those exposed to workplace materials. The MSDS provide information in case of an emergency, such as a child eating a piece of Theraputty. MSDS are not required for personal items stored in handbags or lockers; however, safety is always first, and an OT should not use personal items in clinical use without first addressing all safety issues.

23. Answer: B

Cosigning notes is not evidence of supervision. The OT should maintain a separate logbook whenever the OTA and OT meet to review cases. Answers C and D are incorrect.

24. Answer: D

Rett syndrome is marked by loss of hand skills already acquired in normal development. Choices A, B, and C do not lose hand skills and may or may not have stereotypical hand movements.

25. Answer: D

All are signs, including inability to calm self, clumsiness, poor academic achievement, and delay in speech and language skills.

26. Answer: B

A person with decreased cardiovascular endurance may benefit from aquatic therapy. Choices A, C, and D do not indicate readiness.

27. Answer: A

Hopscotch involves motor synthesis. Answer B is tactile perception, C is cognitive problem-solving and fine motor, and D is visual motor synthesis.

28. Answer: D

Drawing from memory is a visual motor synthesis activity.

29. Answer: C

L. J. King believed that persons with schizophrenia have ineffective proprioceptive feedback mechanisms, an underactive vestibular regulating system, and an inability to fight gravity. Activities should be pleasurable, since thinking about movements tends to slow a person down. Answers A, B, and D all require attention to the movement patterns.

30. Answer: B

A child can maintain head control while supported at 2 months. At 1 month, the child can move his head slightly while in prone. At 4 to 5 months, the child can hold his chest off the floor when in prone.

31. Answer: C

A mature dynamic tripod grasp is typical of a 5- to 6-year-old. A less mature static tripod is used by a 3- to 4-year-old, and the hand moves instead of the fingers during writing. A power grasp is used by a 1-year-old and is fisted with the wrist flexed.

32. Answer: D

ATNR and STNR are brainstem-level reflexes. Parents should understand how reflexes affect function and development; however, the information must be presented in easy-to-understand language.

33. Answer: A

Spasticity is most common and includes hyperactive deep tendon reflexes. Athetoid has varying muscle tone. Atonia is low tone, and mixed is usually spastic with athetoid. Parents can understand the different symptoms to better understand the child's potential.

34. Answer: D

PDDs are distinct from schizophrenia, although children with PDD may occasionally develop schizophrenia later in life. The OTA's function is general education and facilitating a welcoming classroom environment.

35. Answer: C

Occupational therapy practitioners do not advise about medical procedures but may encourage the parent to ask the child's medical staff for advice.

36. Answer: D

As a consultant, you are advising the teacher and the parent. Having the teenager wait until school to shave puts shaving out of the home and into an inappropriate site. Starting a shaving group would only be appropriate if everyone in the class needed instruction, but this is not the case. Currently, the young man has no male role models, as everyone around him of importance is female. A male teenager volunteer could be advised to role model shaving and offer words of encouragement. An electric shaver could provide added safety.

37. Answer: C

Even older adults can improve sensory integration, and being active through life can facilitate this; however, basic SI development is generally developed by age 8 to 10.

38. Answer: C

The client cannot tolerate an upright position and may require a graded program in a reclining back wheelchair. Autonomic dysreflexia is a life-threatening rise in blood pressure with headache and coma; death can occur if untreated. A pulmonary emboli is also life threatening and includes respiratory distress. Answer D is observable in some cases.

39. Answer: A

Suspended equipment, such as swings, is effective in treating vestibular disorders.

40. Answer: A

Scatter rugs are dangerous to everyone. They are often the cause of many home accidents, particularly to those with visual or mobility issues. Scatter rugs are often the cause of falls in the elderly.

41. Answer: D

Often older people lose their sight and do not want to learn braille. The elderly usually prefer to adjust their environment with cues, such as a rubber band on the orange juice but not on the milk.

42. Answer: B

Cross training means that several disciplines can provide for a patient's basic needs. For example, the psychologist can assist the client with using the bathroom, while the OT can assist the client with ambulation.

43. Answer: A

Critical paths or pathways are pre-determined treatment plans for routine treatments. For example, a rehabilitation program may have a critical path for a person with a THR that lays out what is to be reached at days 1, 3, and 5 of rehabilitation. Although critical paths may seem like cookie cutter treatment plans, they are effective in typical patient progress and reduce documentation needs of the OT.

44. Answer: A

Discharge plans are most effective when started at admission. This is true in both medical and psychiatric admissions and provides a focus for the treatment plan.

45. Answer: A

Use of a gentle touch and unhurried motions will reassure the patient.

46. Answer: D

Do not hose a wheelchair with water or let it air dry. Wipe it clean with a metal cleaner available in the car care section of department stores. Do not use light oil on any part of the wheelchair, as it will collect dirt. Use a molybdenum-based grease on the cross brace every 6 months. Educate your patients to follow the owner's manual.

47. Answer: A

People with arthritis often have problems with bathing, and these signs should not be confused with dementia. Answers B, C, and D have issues with ADLs in general, not just bathing.

48. Answer: B

All are signs of EPS except the inability to sustain tongue movements. EPS includes increased movement of the tongue, both in and out of the mouth. In addition, EPS can include jaw biting, clenching, chewing, or mouth opening.

49. Answer: B

Have the client repeat information back by asking, "We have covered a lot of information today. Can you summarize all the important information for me?" Always use the word medicine instead of pills or drugs. Avoid technical words altogether, and never change the medication bottles. If the client is having a hard time with the bottles, encourage the client to ask the pharmacist to change the bottles for him or her.

50. Answer: B

Elderly that are cognitively impaired, such as those with dementia, do well in structured programs with activities; however, too many choices can be confusing. Validating feelings can greatly reduce anxiety. Names and pictures on doors help the resident find his or her room.

Section Two

1. Which of the following alternatives to restraints for the wandering elderly is *not* effective?
   A. Opportunity for exercise
   B. Put bells on their shoes
   C. Safe, closed area outside or inside
   D. Identity bracelet

2. Activities that are alerting to the sensory integrative systems include all of the following *except*:
   A. Fast, loud music of variable intensity
   B. Swinging or sustained movements
   C. Light touch, whisking, brushing movements
   D. Increased muscle activities

3. The OTA should look for feeding issues when addressing ADLs. All of the following are common pathological causes of feeding and swallowing disorders in the elderly *except*:
   A. Stroke
   B. Head trauma
   C. Liver or kidney disease
   D. Degenerative neurological disorders

4. For maximum support and comfort, the length of a forearm splint should be how long?
   A. One-fourth of the forearm
   B. One-third of the forearm
   C. One-half of the forearm
   D. Two-thirds of the forearm

5. Drug reactions are common in the elderly. What statement is *not* true about medication reactions in older adults?
   A. Toxic reactions can occur with low drug dosages
   B. Reactions can include drowsiness, depression, confusion, or dizziness
   C. Medications can cause involuntary movements or drug-related parkinsonism
   D. Over-the-counter drugs, such as antacids, cold medicines, and laxatives, are safe

6. Alternatives to restraining elderly residents who are unsteady on their feet include all of the following *except*:
   A. Address possible low vision problems
   B. Reading material or books on tapes
   C. Soft slippers and increased ambulation
   D. Meaningful activities in which to participate

7. Activities that are calming to the sensory integrative systems include all of the following *except*:
   A. Defy gravity, up and down
   B. Swinging or sustained movements
   C. Heavy touch, massage
   D. Decreased motor activities

8. All of the following techniques are effective in the behavioral management of persons with brain injury *except*:

   A. Praise efforts of the client to regain control

   B. Give an alternative, such as, "I'll have to report this behavior to the team"

   C. Create a plan or agreement to accomplish tasks

   D. Ignore negative, attention-seeking behaviors and comments

9. OTAs need to be aware of epilepsy as a secondary diagnosis to several disabilities. At what age is the highest frequency of epilepsy seen?

   A. Birth to 10

   B. 11 to 39

   C. 40 to 69

   D. 70+

10. What would be the *best* treatment option for a child with sensory integration, particularly vestibular, problems?

   A. Reading a book in a big, overstuffed chair in the library

   B. Playing on the fixed monkey bars in the school yard

   C. Playing on the swing set in the school yard

   D. Being wrapped up tight in a blanket in a comfortably warm room

11. All of the following statements are true concerning phantom sensation following limb loss in adults *except*:

   A. Almost all adults experience phantom sensations following limb loss

   B. 60% of all patients experience phantom pain

   C. Phantom pain is considered a disturbance in body image

   D. The existence of neurological scheme ends with the actual physical loss of the limb

12. A patient with left-sided hemiplegia is asked to draw a clock. All of the following are being evaluated *except*:

   A. Visual perception

   B. Visual sequencing

   C. Visual constructive ability

   D. Ability to tell time

13. The medical doctor has stopped the OTA to ask a question about a patient's weekly progress note that uses the words "gradations of activities." The doctor is unclear and would like further clarification. Gradation of an activity means:

   A. Assigning a grade to the patient's completed task

   B. Adjusting the pace and modifying the demand to meet the patient's maximum capabilities

   C. Assigning minimal to maximum assistance to the task depending on the amount of assistance the patient needs from the OTA

   D. Encouraging the patient to try one more time to complete an uncompleted task

14. All of the following demonstrate good listening skills *except*:

   A. Lean slightly backward

   B. Make eye contact

   C. Body appears open

   D. Face client squarely

Use the following information to answer questions 15, 16, 17, and 18.

You are an occupational therapy practitioner working in a specialized facility for people with head traumas. Your facility treats clients from subacute to community re-entry and outpatient. The facility uses RLA levels to assign clients to different programs. You have clients in all the different programs.

15. When working with patients with head injuries, at what level does sensory stimulation treatment seem *most* appropriate?
    A. Level I
    B. Level III
    C. Level V
    D. Level VII

16. When would the same sensory stimulation treatment be the *most* inappropriate?
    A. Level I
    B. Level II
    C. Level III
    D. Level IV

17. At what level is repetition and practice of tasks *most* appropriate?
    A. Level IV
    B. Level V
    C. Level VI
    D. Level VII

18. Level VIII is purposeful and appropriate interaction with the environment. All of the following would be effective treatment for a client at level VIII *except*:
    A. Cognitive rehabilitation
    B. Vocational rehabilitation
    C. Work hardening programs
    D. Community mobility training

19. The *best* response to a person who is clearly psychotic, telling you how the FBI and CIA are chasing him, is:
    A. "I have to go now"
    B. "That's very interesting. Tell me more about that"
    C. "Now think about this, you know it can't be true. It's part of your disease"
    D. "That sounds crazy to me. I can't talk to you when you say these things"

20. What activity is *most* appropriate for a person hearing threatening voices?
    A. A 1,000-piece puzzle
    B. A tie-dyed t-shirt
    C. Leather wallet with written directions
    D. Learning a simple word processing computer program

21. People with Parkinson's disease are often given medication that is dopamine-based, which improves movement. However, as dopamine increases, what side effect also increases?

    A. Cog wheel movements

    B. Unsteady gait

    C. Psychotic features

    D. Confusion

22. People usually do not realize this, but most human beings hold their breath when they bend over to pick up something, tie their shoe, or garden. What population is this particularly dangerous to?

    A. Cardiac patients

    B. Multiple sclerosis patients

    C. Those with orthopedic conditions

    D. Arthritis patients

23. At the end of your treatment session with a client, she begins to cry, stating, "I've just been diagnosed with epilepsy. The kids at school will think I'm a freak." After using your counseling skills to reassure the client, you provide her with general information about epilepsy. The approximate percentage of individuals with epilepsy that can be successfully treated with anti-epileptic medications is:

    A. 10%

    B. 50%

    C. 80%

    D. 100%

24. Aquatic therapy has positive effects on function. The primary principle of this modality is buoyancy. If your 42-year-old patient with head trauma weighs 220 pounds on land, what is his approximate weight in the water?

    A. 220 pounds

    B. 175 pounds

    C. 110 pounds

    D. 75 pounds

25. AOTPAC is the political action committee that represents the profession of occupational therapy. AOTPAC suggests all occupational therapists must take an active role in national legislation that affects occupational therapy. When writing a letter to your congress person or your senator:

    A. Explain how the issue will impact you and your community

    B. Avoid form letters

    C. Be constructive in your proposals, offering professional advice

    D. All of the above

26. You are about to treat a patient bedside but "Methicillin Resistant Staphylococcus Aureus" (MRSA) is noted in his chart. What does this mean?

    A. The patient is an IV abusing or recreational drug user

    B. The patient is ventilator dependent and requires oxygen monitoring

    C. The patient has an infection that cannot be treated with traditional antibiotics

    D. The patient is HIV positive and requires the use of universal precautions

27. If assessment on the Baltimore Therapeutic Equipment (BTE) simulator suggests that the maximum a female workers' compensation client can lift at this time is 7 pounds, what item in her home will she be *unable* to lift?

    A. A jumbo box of cereal

    B. A gallon of milk

    C. A blow dryer

    D. A portable telephone

28. Understanding an individual's weight-bearing precautions is essential to addressing mobility with a client. What level allows a small amount of weight to be applied by the affected leg?

    A. Toe-touch weight-bearing (TTWB)

    B. Partial weight-bearing (PWB)

    C. Weight-bearing as tolerated (WBAT)

    D. Full weight-bearing (FWB)

29. An entry-level OTA with less than 1 year of experience must have close supervision by an OT or intermediate/advanced OTA. How is close supervision defined?

    A. Constant, direct supervision of all treatment sessions

    B. Daily, direct contact at the work site

    C. Direct contact at least every 2 weeks with telephone contact more often

    D. Direct contact once a month with telephone contact as needed

30. When a person suspected of having Alzheimer's disease cannot handle his finances but is still able to handle a demanding work schedule, what differential diagnosis might be present?

    A. Other forms of dementia in addition to Alzheimer's disease

    B. Pseudodementia due to depression

    C. CVA

    D. Anoxia from COPD

31. What over-the-counter medications are contraindicated for a person in cardiac rehabilitation?

    A. Vitamins

    B. Aspirin

    C. Tylenol brand pain relievers

    D. Alka Seltzer brand stomach and cold remedies

32. What law specifically prohibits discrimination based solely on an individual's disability in any program receiving federal monies?

    A. Rehabilitation Act of 1973, Section 504

    B. Education of the Handicapped Act

    C. ADA

    D. PL 94-103

33. Vertical righting reactions in children:

    A. Activate muscles to move the midline of the body into alignment with the center of gravity

    B. Activate muscles to lift the head to either side

    C. Are present at birth

    D. All of the above

34. When a child is supported in the supine position and his head is gently dropped, what reflex elicits abduction and extension of the arms followed by the arms coming together in an arc?
    A. Flexor withdrawal
    B. Crossed extension
    C. Moro's
    D. Bauer's

35. The OTA has been asked to join a committee to develop a new program for community outreach. The OTA's assigned task is to check for documents that define OT roles. The OTA has checked with state licensure agencies and has been referred to AOTA. AOTA defines an occupational therapy practitioner as:
    A. An OT
    B. An OT and OTA
    C. An OT, OTA, or OT aide
    D. Any person who practices occupational therapy

36. The *Occupational Therapy Roles* paper is an official document of the AOTA. What roles are defined in this document?
    A. OT and OTA practitioners
    B. Clinical and education fieldwork educators
    C. Supervisor, administrator, consultant, and entrepreneur
    D. All of the above

37. What factor is *most* important in patient compliance with splint usage after discharge?
    A. Adjust the splint in response to the patient's complaints
    B. Have the patient practice putting on and taking off the splint
    C. Label the splint for correct usage
    D. Contrast the colors of the splint and the straps

38. An 88-year-old nursing home resident is 7 years post-CVA. Her left hand is fisted, and passive ROM is painful to her. What is the *best* intervention?
    A. None; leave the situation alone
    B. Daily soaks in warm water to keep her hand clean
    C. Resting hand splint
    D. Soft splint

39. What is the *first* thing an OTA should do when washing her hands?
    A. Turn on the water and adjust the temperature
    B. Apply soap to her hands
    C. Remove rings and put them on the sink's edge
    D. Pull out a length of paper towel

40. An OTA is anticipating the opening of a new dementia unit in the skilled nursing home at which she works The purpose of the unit is to provide assessment and referral for the appropriate level of care from returning to independence to 24-hour nursing care. The OTA wants to assess both performance areas and components as they relate to ADLs. What assessment would be *best*?

    A. Allen's Cognitive Levels

    B. Cognitive Performance Test

    C. Kohlman Evaluation of Living Skills

    D. Mini-Mental Status Exam

41. In what position should the neck be splinted for a pediatric patient with burns?

    A. 10 degrees hyperextension

    B. 10 degrees flexion

    C. Flexion as much as possible

    D. 0 degrees, neutral

42. A hyperactive gag reflex may be normalized by:

    A. Icing the lips and having the patient say "OOO"

    B. Offering resistance to opening the jaw

    C. Walking a tongue depressor toward the back of the tongue

    D. Sucking through a 6-inch straw and gradually increasing the straw length

43. If a patient slightly cuts his finger while cutting vegetables in the ADL kitchen, the OTA should follow universal precautions and then:

    A. Call a medical emergency

    B. Hand the patient a gauze, and ask him to apply pressure to the cut

    C. Call his nurse to the kitchen

    D. Call the OT supervisor for assistance

44. Quality assurance (QA) requires the development of indicators as variables that indicate quality care of the patient. All of the following would be appropriate occupational therapy indicators in a mental health service *except*:

    A. OT assessment initiated within 24 hours of admission

    B. QA plan will be monitored monthly

    C. Patient involvement in goal setting is indicated by patient signature on the OT treatment plan

    D. Documentation of progress follows facility rules

45. Your client is complaining his wheelchair is too tight. When measuring for his wheelchair, what consideration should be made for the seat?

    A. None; the seat is standard, so no measurements are needed

    B. If doorways in the patient's home are narrow, the wheelchair seat must be narrow

    C. Seat should be 4 inches wider than the patient's widest point across his hips or thighs, so he can move around easier

    D. Seat should be 2 inches wider than the patient's widest point across his hips or thighs. If braces are worn, width should be increased

46. A confused head-injured patient may ask a lot of questions, often repeating the same question over and over. What is the *best* activity for this patient?

    A. Nothing; the patient is too agitated; he needs quiet

    B. Socializing with other patients

    C. Looking at his memory book

    D. Playing cards

47. Vestibular stimulation can be used to increase muscle tone in both adults and children. Always watch the patient for emotional reactions. Spinning should *not* be done with what type of person?

    A. Persons over the age of 50

    B. Persons with poor ROM

    C. Persons prone to seizures

    D. Persons who are 6 feet or taller in height

48. Spina bifida is a disorder characterized by failure of the vertebral column to close. Children may have a shunt placed in their heads. All of the following are warning signs of a malfunctioning shunt *except*:

    A. Irritability and fussiness

    B. Vomiting

    C. Headache

    D. Wide open eyes, iris is totally visible

49. The ADA has had sweeping reforms in barrier-free designs. When planning the floor space of any treatment area, what is the minimum width of a door frame?

    A. 28 inches

    B. 30 inches

    C. 32 inches

    D. 36 inches

50. Occupational therapy departments should develop departmental policies for all of the following reasons *except*:

    A. Policies clarify prohibited behaviors

    B. Policies negate the *Code of Ethics*

    C. Policies are guides to thinking and action

    D. Policies suggest courses of action

Section Two Answers and Explanations

1. Answer: B
Wandering elderly are often confused as well. Bells on their shoes may act as an alarm but not likely. A safe inside environment and a closed outside environment allows wandering without danger.

2. Answer: B
Mildred Ross describes this as a calming activity.

3. Answer: C
Liver or kidney disease may affect the patient's interest in food, diet requirements, or digestion but does not affect swallowing.

4. Answer: D
The forearm will be more comfortable with support of two-thirds its length.

5. Answer: D
Over-the-counter medicines can also cause adverse drug reactions, especially when mixed with prescriptions. The longer an individual is on a medication, the greater the likelihood of drug reactions. Drugs are a major cause of dizziness in persons over age 60.

6. Answer: C
Increased ambulation does improve unsteadiness, but appropriate footwear that provides support must be worn. Answers A, B, and D provide additional alternatives to restraints.

7. Answer: A
Mildred Ross describes this as an alerting activity.

8. Answer: B
This approach is evidence of a power struggle and is often perceived as threatening by the patient who can easily become defensive. Answers A, C, and D are all behavioral techniques aimed at increasing positive reinforcement to increase desired behaviors.

9. Answer: A
Newborns to youth have the highest frequency of epilepsy. Numbers decrease in the 11- to 70-year-old age range and increase again at age 70 due to increased health problems and medications.

10. Answer: C
Vestibular treatment with swings or suspended equipment is most effective, although the fixed monkey bars may be able to provide some movement. Answers A and D provide no movement and, therefore, no treatment; however, they are likely to be preferred by a child with vestibular problems.

11. Answer: D
Almost all adults experience some sensation, with over half experiencing pain. Phantom pain does disturb body image but may aid in rehabilitation in that the patient continues to have body perception during training. Phantom pain exists because the neurological scheme continues after loss of the actual limb.

12. Answer: D
The clock drawing task is a non-standardized but effective tool to evaluate perceptual problems often seen in those people with CVAs and left-sided weakness. The task is perceptual, not cognitive, and does not evaluate the ability to tell time.

13. Answer: B

Gradation is adapting an activity higher or lower to provide adequate challenge but guarantee success in the patient. All other answers are false.

14. Answer: A

Good listening skills include all of the answers except the therapist should lean slightly forward toward the client. Facing the client, maintaining eye contact, and appearing relaxed and open tells the client, "I'm here for you."

15. Answer: A

Level I, no response, and Level II, generalized response, are appropriate for sensory stimulation. Level III, localized response, may further benefit, but they can begin to handle other activities.

16. Answer: D

Level IV, confused agitated, is a heightened state of activity with agitation. Sensory stimulation would not be appropriate for this client, as it would likely confuse him or her more.

17. Answer: C

Level VI is the confused but appropriate level, where clients benefit from repetition and practice in a safe environment. The levels before VI are confused, inappropriate or agitated, and tasks may not be practiced successfully. Level VII is community-based because practice is in the community.

18. Answer: A

Cognitive rehabilitation is most heavy in levels V and VI with complex tasks managed at level VII. Level VIII would have mastered the skills.

19. Answer: B

Leaving or confronting a delusional person isolates the person. Delusions are unreal beliefs that cannot be cleared with facts. Until the person's thoughts clear with medication, the best approach is to validate the person's feelings without feeding into the delusion.

20. Answer: B

Answers A, C, and D require too much attention for this patient to successfully complete. The tie-dyed t-shirt is a success-oriented project. Even if mistakes are made because the client is distracted, the shirt will usually come out well.

21. Answer: C

This side effect makes sense if you think about two diseases, Parkinson's and schizophrenia. People with Parkinson's disease have decreased levels of dopamine, and people with schizophrenia have too much dopamine. As the medication increases to improve movement, psychotic features may present.

22. Answer: A

Bending over is a concern for all the diagnoses listed, but holding the breath while bending over is of particular danger for cardiac patients, as the two combined adds additional stress on the heart.

23. Answer: C

According to data collected in 1996, 80% of all people with epilepsy can be successfully treated. Although the disease is not cured, medication can reduce seizure activity, modifying the disease process to reduce further damage to the CNS.

24. Answer: C

The biomechanical frame of reference shows that the buoyancy of water supports half of the body weight.

25. Answer: D

When writing legislative letters, include all of the items, as well as address the letter correctly, keep comments to the point, and be respectful.

26. Answer: C

All of the items are false except C. It is important that the OT be aware of MRSA because the therapist is at risk of becoming infected or passing the infection on to others. Follow hospital guidelines for gowning, wearing gloves, and wearing eye protection.

27. Answer: B

A gallon of milk weighs over 8 pounds (128 ounces/16 ounces per pound = 8 pounds plus the container weight). All the other items weigh about 2 pounds.

28. Answer: B

TTWB does not allow any weight but allows the toe to be used for balance. WBAT allows weight to be applied until pain. FWB has no restrictions.

29. Answer: B

A new graduate OTA must be supervised at the site with daily direct contact. Intermediate or advanced OTAs can have routine or general supervision.

30. Answer: B

Depression is likely the cause. All the other diagnoses would have additional signs.

31. Answer: D

The high level of sodium of these products should not be used with cardiac clients. The OTA should advise the client to not use this product until cleared by the medical doctor.

32. Answer: A

All the acts have influenced the education of children in the United States. Section 504 specifically states programs receive federal monies. This is one of the reasons college campuses have Section 504 coordinators, so any student on campus can qualify for financial aid programs.

33. Answer: A

Vertical righting reactions include body righting. They are not present at birth but develop with interaction with the environment. Turning the head is part of rotational righting reactions.

34. Answer: C

Flexor withdrawal, crossed extension, and Bauer's are all reflexes tested with touch pressure to the foot.

35. Answer: B

OT practitioners are OTs and OTAs who are certified to practice. OT aides or technicians require intense, close supervision by the OT and/or OTA.

36. Answer: D

In addition, the paper also describes the roles of faculty, program director, researcher, and scholar.

37. Answer: A

Compliance for all treatments is improved when the OTA listens to the patient's issues. Answers B, C, and D may also be useful in treatment.

38. Answer: D

A soft splint, such as a palm protector, can assist in skin hygiene and improve quality of life without the added discomfort caused by a rigid hand splint.

39. Answer: D

Pull out a length of towels to have ready when washing hands, turn on the water, and adjust. Apply soap to hands with rings on, and wash completely. Rinse hands and leave water running. Dry hands with the towel, and use the towel to turn off the water.

40. Answer: C

The KELS is a measure of performance areas. The other three assessments are appropriate for dementia but measure cognitive performance components.

41. Answer: D

The neck should be in neutral.

42. Answer: C

Walking the tongue depressor toward the back of the tongue will desensitize the gag reflex. The patient should control the tongue depressor when possible while the therapist observes. Icing is an exercise for muscle strength. Resistance to the jaw is for jaw control. Increasing the straw length is effective for the sucking reflex.

43. Answer: B

If possible, have the patient apply pressure himself. If not, the OT should don a latex glove, put a gauze on the cut, and apply pressure. Return the patient to his unit and notify the nurse. Fill out the appropriate incident report forms.

44. Answer: B

This is a monitoring plan. Choices A, C, and D are all indicators of quality programs.

45. Answer: D

Two inches wider than the user is correct. One size does not fit all, and too much padding or room can cause sores.

46. Answer: C

The OTA could make a memory book for the patient that includes answers to common questions like, "Where am I?" Include family pictures and reality orientation information. Keep the book simple to reduce agitation and light in case the patient should throw it. Having the patient play cards or socialize with others may be too much stimulation. Doing nothing is likely to get the patient more agitated.

47. Answer: C

Spinning is contraindicated for people prone to seizures.

48. Answer: D

Irritability, vomiting, headaches, and "setting sun" eyes (partially visible irises) are all symptoms of a malfunctioning shunt.

49. Answer: C

The width of the door opening should be a minimum of 32 inches.

50. Answer: B

The *Code of Ethics* cannot be altered. Answers A, C, and D are all true.

Section Three

1. At the end of a group in the arts and crafts room of a locked psychiatric hospital, the OTA finds that a pair of scissors is missing. The *first* thing the OTA should do is:

   A. Walk around the room to see if the scissors are visible

   B. Walk around the room and ask everyone if they have the scissors

   C. Stand by the door and ask everyone if they have the scissors

   D. Initiate the dangerous instrument search procedure

2. A female patient is admitted to an inpatient psychiatric facility for a 3-day evaluation after police were called to her home on a domestic disturbance call. When the police arrived, the couple was involved in a physical and verbal fight. The husband was intoxicated and was sent for a 3-day evaluation to another facility. During the first 2 days, the female patient was going to leave her husband, but now she is crying and saying how much she misses her "love." What should the OTA do?

   A. Model separateness and encourage the patient to develop boundaries

   B. Educate the patient to domestic violence

   C. Inform the patient that this new behavior is not healthy

   D. Ignore the negative behavior and focus attention elsewhere

3. The OTA in a community mental health program based on the Fountain House Model has been approached by the consumers to lead a group on alternative treatment techniques. The OTA has only basic understanding of alternative treatments. What is the *best* response?

   A. The OTA should discourage the idea because of the possible conflicts with the consumers' current treatment

   B. The OTA should acknowledge the request but ask for time to research the topics

   C. The OTA should tell the consumers that she has no information or training in this area and refer the consumers to an alternative treatment specialist

   D. The OTA should tell the consumers that she has no information or training in this area and refer the consumers to their medical doctors

4. An elderly woman recently admitted to a nursing home has become depressed and is refusing to leave her room. She is eating only minimal food. Her family and doctor have agreed to begin anti-depressive medication. The nursing staff has referred the resident to the OT/OTA team for evaluation and treatment. The COPM was used for the evaluation, but the OT feels the client is too depressed and not accurately reporting her issues. What should the OTA do *next*?

   A. Wait the 10 days that typically are needed for the resident to feel the effects of the medication, then ask the OT to give the COPM again

   B. Ask the nursing staff to get the patient out of bed and in a wheelchair. Take the resident on a tour of the OT department

   C. Make a short appointment with the resident during lunch, and sit and talk with her

   D. Bring an animal-assisted therapy pet to her room and offer to let her pet it

5. The parents of a 26-year-old male would like their son to move out on his own so they can sell their home and move to their retirement home in another state. The parents are very concerned that their son have a supported home life with continued services in the community mental health program in which he is currently participating. The OT/OTA team is asked to evaluate the client and make recommendations. After using the KELS, ACL, and a home visit, it is clear the client does not have the skills to be independent in the community. The client wants his own apartment if he cannot live with his parents. What should the OT/OTA team do *first*?

    A. Arrange a meeting with the parents and the client to discuss future plans

    B. Talk with the client about the evaluation findings and ask if a meeting can be set up with the parents

    C. Let the parents know the evaluation results, find out their time line for selling the house, and begin ADL and IADL training

    D. Refer the client to a housing specialist who can arrange a supportive housing system

6. A person with a 20-year history of schizophrenia has learned that there are numerous jobs for people with computer skills. She would like to learn word processing because she "used to be good at typing." What should the OTA do *first*?

    A. Place her in front of a computer and give her basic, simple instructions. Observe how she handles the situation

    B. Talk to her about her lack of general job skills and inability to hold other more basic jobs in the past

    C. Talk to her about her past work experience and current motivations for a word processing job

    D. Set up an appointment with the client for a work evaluation and see how she does

7. The OTA and therapeutic recreator are taking a group of seniors from a long-term psychiatric unit on a short hike to a picnic area. All the participants have been medically cleared for this activity. Nursing has provided sunscreen, bug repellent, and hats for the hikers. What other issue is *most* important?

    A. Appropriate social behavior

    B. Long pants to avoid tick or bug bites

    C. Medication that is typically given during meals

    D. Hydration

8. During a team meeting, a client who keeps fainting is discussed. The client is on several psychiatric medications, but evaluation of the medication has shown these are not the cause of the fainting. The client's vital signs are normal. Several staff feel the client is simply exaggerating lightheadedness to get staff's attention. The OTA has noticed the fainting seems to happen more with activity than when staying still. The OTA suspects possible:

    A. Blood pressure problems

    B. Anxiety and hyperventilation

    C. Migraines

    D. Vestibular disorder

9. A couple dealing with the early to middle stages of Alzheimer's disease has decided that the person with the disease will remain at home as long as possible. The OTA has recommended all of the following safety adjustments to the home *except*:

    A. Place a deadbolt on the front door

    B. Cover the cellar door with a sheet

    C. Remove the lock on the bathroom door

    D. Remove the stoppers on the sinks and tubs

10. An OTA with less than 1 year experience has joined an OT department with 11 other OTs and OTAs. The department manager wants to facilitate everyone's professional development, so he has randomly assigned each person a month when they will present a 45-minute inservice on the topic of their choice related to work. The new OTA is assigned next month's inservice and does not want to do this because she is new. What should the managing OT do?

    A. Give the new OTA a different month so she has more experience

    B. Have the new OTA keep the inservice date. Encourage the new OT to present a new topic learned in school

    C. Excuse the new OTA from the inservice because she is new to the job

    D. Have the new OTA keep the inservice date and learn a topic in the next month

11. Adults recovering from burns and wearing pressure garments often complain of all of the following *except*:

    A. Skin itchiness

    B. Limb swelling

    C. Cut-off blood circulation

    D. Skin tenderness

12. The provision of education and instruction to consumers of work injury prevention can include all of the following *except*:

    A. Medical diagnosis

    B. Stress management

    C. Proper body mechanics

    D. Postural awareness

13. An OTA is working with a woman with a CVA. Nursing has stated that the patient sometimes has difficulty with some foods and not others. The OTA is concerned with:

    A. Compensatory swallowing techniques

    B. Positioning

    C. Thermal stimulation

    D. Grading or altering the bolus

14. A slanted surface for a lap tray or desktop provides:

    A. Forearm support

    B. Increased fatigue

    C. Increased extraneous movements

    D. Decreased hand tremors

15. When using cooking as a modality with a client with aphasia, what is the *first* step?

    A. Use a recipe from a recipe book of the client's choice

    B. Use a boxed mix that contains most of the needed ingredients

    C. Make gelatin or pudding from a box

    D. Make familiar recipes known by heart

16. What technique allows one-handed cooks additional function without adaptive equipment?

    A. Home companion

    B. Sitting while preparing food

    C. Photo cookbook

    D. Forearm support

17. What work adaptation is *most* appropriate in reducing back pressure for a computer operator?
    A. Slanted foot stool
    B. High-back chair
    C. High arm rests
    D. Posture support belt

18. What technique is *most* effective in assessing muscle strength in a home care client?
    A. MMT
    B. Cybex machine
    C. ROM
    D. Functional strength pattern testing

19. What is the *most* effective method to note the presence of tone in a client?
    A. PROM, quickly
    B. PROM, slowly
    C. Active assistive range of motion (AAROM), quickly
    D. AAROM, slowly

20. How should a person with arthritis be taught to open a jar?
    A. Rubber grip, turning to the ulnar side
    B. Rubber grip, turning to the radial side
    C. Dishcloth grip, turning to the ulnar side
    D. Dishcloth grip, turning to the radial side

21. What activity is *best* in encouraging co-contraction in children with low tone?
    A. Playing statue
    B. Going through an obstacle course
    C. Pretending to ice skate around the room
    D. Finger painting

22. SOAP notes are sometimes used for documentation. Your patient has just told you that he is upset with how his treatment is progressing. In what section would the patient's comments go?
    A. Subjective (S)
    B. Objective (O)
    C. Assessment (A)
    D. Plan (P)

23. What factor is *most* important in OT staff retention?
    A. High salaries
    B. Job satisfaction
    C. Continuing education opportunities
    D. Health insurance benefits

24. Research and evidence-based practice in occupational therapy is:
    A. Well-developed and complete
    B. Usually done with other disciplines
    C. In the early stages of growth and development
    D. Of little value because it is statistical in nature

25. Your client is a 6-year-old boy who is highly distracted. You have designed a very structured program aimed at providing a successful experience for the patient. Your environment should be:
    A. Bright colors with several choices of toys for fine motor skill development
    B. Distracting, competitive stimuli has been reduced
    C. A simulated classroom
    D. No particular environmental factors need to be addressed due to the structured program

26. The OTA/OT team has been asked to join a committee to begin planning a new occupational therapy clinic after a major donor has given the department grant funds to update the appearance. Capital expenses of an occupational therapy program might include:
    A. Land and buildings
    B. Supplies
    C. Equipment under $500.00
    D. OT staff salaries

27. Doorknobs should be placed at what height from the floor to allow for accessibility by people in wheelchairs?
    A. 28 inches
    B. 30 inches
    C. 32 inches
    D. 36 inches

28. The format for documentation is largely:
    A. Decided by management at the facility
    B. Agreed upon by majority rule within the OT department
    C. Outlined by regulation or law
    D. Developed by faculty from OT schools

29. Certification of an OTA is granted by:
    A. AOTA, AMA, and APA jointly
    B. OTA's own association
    C. State certification boards
    D. NBCOT

30. Your client is a 4-year-old girl with CP and very low tone. When she is positioned in her customized wheelchair, her head is forward and she cannot maintain the vertical position. What is the *best* intervention?
    A. Recline the wheelchair so gravity will pull her head into neutral
    B. Give verbal commands to pull up her head
    C. Present an object in her visual field to elicit extension through eye tracking
    D. Use a soft cervical collar or molded neck collar to increase head control

31. The mother of a 5-year-old child with developmental delays tells you that she is unable to do his home care program because she is "too busy." You suspect there might be other reasons. What should you do *first*?

    A. Emphasize the importance of the home program

    B. Discontinue the program and see the client in the clinic again

    C. Talk to the mother about problems she is facing

    D. Provide more information on how to make the home program easier

32. During an OT task group, you observe your patient's cognitive abilities. Henry is able to complete a simple three-step craft project with visual cueing at each step from the OTA. While disregarding the written directions, Henry uses the sample project as a guide but uses too much glue. His attention span is intact for 45 minutes. Besides a simple craft project, what other activity would be *best* for Henry to work on cognitive functioning?

    A. Use a bus schedule

    B. Make a sandwich

    C. Budgeting for 1 day

    D. Make a craft kit that snaps together

33. An OTA is asked to give a presentation to a local advocacy group for adults with mental health problems. The *most* effective presentation would be:

    A. Reviewing assessments such as BaFPE, ACL, and KELS

    B. Discussing problems that adults with mental health diagnosis might have and how occupational therapy addresses the problems

    C. A demonstration of new computer programs to refer patients to community placements

    D. Teach basic counseling techniques so the audience can use them with its consumers

34. What governmental program provides medical coverage for people age 65 and over?

    A. Medicaid

    B. Medicare

    C. Social security insurance (SSI)/social security disability (SSD)

    D. Welfare and Section 8

35. The purpose of documentation includes all of the following *except*:

    A. Data for research, education, reimbursement, treatment

    B. Serial and legal record of therapeutic intervention

    C. Facilitate communication among health care professionals

    D. Cover the therapist in case there is an ethical problem

36. What activity is *best* for encouraging the integration of primitive postural reflexes in a child?

    A. Have the child lie prone on a scooter board and spin

    B. Have the child walk on a balance beam

    C. Have the child pretend to be a dog, crawl around, roll over, and bark

    D. Have the child play a game of marbles

37. The NBCOT registration exam can be taken:

    A. After all classwork is finished

    B. After all fieldwork is finished

    C. After all classwork and fieldwork are finished

    D. After licensure is filed for

38. Vestibular stimulation when used to treat a child with autism is *least* effective for improving which of the following?

    A. Communication

    B. Hypo-responsiveness

    C. Self-care

    D. Muscle tone

39. Your 5-year-old patient is coming to OT to inhibit tonic neck reflex and to increase tolerance to vestibular stimulation. You ask the child to roll in a carpeted barrel or innertube with handles. What precaution is *most* important?

    A. Be aware that others watching will think the activity is unsafe

    B. Be aware that children may think of the barrel as a weapon

    C. Be aware of too much pressure on the child's hips and legs

    D. Be aware of too much vestibular input and the emotional responses

40. You hear a group of therapists talking about types of documentation and their favorites. What does POMR stand for?

    A. Problem-oriented medical record

    B. Performance-oriented medical record

    C. Problem observation medical record

    D. Patient-oriented medical record

41. Your client has an above-the-knee amputation. What issue is *most* important in teaching ADLs?

    A. Use of adaptive equipment

    B. How to supervise others who help with home management

    C. Energy conservation and work simplification

    D. Cognitive retraining

42. Your client is a 12-month-old girl who exhibits poor integration of primitive reflexes with impaired hand-to-mouth and hand-to-body movements. What would be the *best* intervention by OT?

    A. Rolling, pushing up on extended elbows from a prone position

    B. Visual tracking of a toy to increase eye ROM

    C. Reaching for a toy to improve eye-hand coordination

    D. Moving small pegs from cup to cup

43. Which of the following activities is *best* for a client with dissociative disorder (multiple personality disorder) whose goal is to increase self-awareness and express her feelings?

    A. Horticulture

    B. Arts and crafts

    C. Sports

    D. Art therapy

Use the following information to answer questions 44 and 45:

Another occupational therapy practitioner has told you during lunch that he is really behind in his billable units for the week, so he is going to bill patients for the time this week and make up for it next week.

44. This breaks what section of the AOTA *Code of Ethics*?
    A. Principle 1, beneficence
    B. Principle 2, nonmaleficence
    C. Principle 3, autonomy, privacy, confidentiality
    D. Principle 4, duties

45. The *best* response after telling the practitioner that this is illegal is:
    A. Notify the billing department that false billing has occurred
    B. Notify the area coordinator that there is a problem in the department
    C. Speak to the therapist privately and tell him that this is unethical
    D. Report the unethical behavior to the ethics committee of the AOTA

46. What factor is *least* effective in developing a bowel program for a person with a SCI?
    A. Timing and a regular schedule
    B. Hot liquid intake or light snack
    C. Suppository use or digital stimulation
    D. At the convenience of the person

47. Your client is a 19-year-old male recovering from a TBI as a result of speeding his car late at night. He is doing well in his rehabilitation. Friends have been visiting lately and are motivating him by saying there will be a big "bash" for him when he is discharged. Your client keeps talking about the party and how he cannot wait to have a beer. You have counseled him about the use of alcohol and drugs after a TBI, and he and his family understand this, but they want to know "How much is okay?" You respond:
    A. Limit one drink per day
    B. 3 to 4 months post-injury
    C. 2 years post-injury
    D. Never drink again

48. An OTA working on a medical rehabilitation unit must be aware of heterotopic ossification in patients due to lack of movement. What diagnosis is *least* likely to develop this condition?
    A. SCI
    B. Guillain-Barré syndrome
    C. Burns
    D. Multiple sclerosis

49. An OTA working on a SCI unit is likely to hear what complaint *most* often?
    A. Fatigue
    B. Spasticity
    C. Depression
    D. Bowel control and cleaning

50. An OTA wants to take patients with mental health disabilities outside for a game of volleyball. Besides hydration, what special issue do people on psychotropic medications have?
    A. Sensitivity to light
    B. Sunburn easily
    C. Get muscle cramps easily
    D. Fatigue quickly

Section Three Answers and Explanations

1. Answer: C
If the clients were allowed in the arts and crafts room, they are likely to have behavior that excuses initiating the dangerous sharps policy immediately. The OTA should, for safety, position herself between the clients and the door and ask for the missing scissors. Likely, the sharps were simply misplaced and will be found immediately. If not, the OTA should call for assistance.

2. Answer: A
The OTA should model separateness, healthy expression, and boundaries because the client is currently dealing with co-dependency issues and does not know how to behave as a separate individual in a relationship. Education about violence can be helpful only after a person sees the reality of the relationship. Ignoring the behavior can be appropriate in a behavioral conditioning frame of reference but not likely effective in short-term acute evaluation.

3. Answer: B
The OTA should acknowledge her lack of current information but should seek information from both alternative medicine resources and opposing scientific sources. Some alternative treatments are helpful in conjunction with medical treatment, and some simply have no scientific proof or are contraindicated. The informed consumer can make informed decisions.

4. Answer: D
The resident is sending a clear message that she does not want human contact. Despite knowing this is not healthy, relationships cannot be forced. A pet introduced to the resident (if she accepts) is the logical next activity to try. An animal-assisted trained dog might be brought to her bedside to see if she will pet it. A small lap pet, such as a bunny, might also be tried.

5. Answer: B
The client is a legal adult, and the OTA needs to have his permission to talk to the parent unless the parent maintains guardianship. Once permission is obtained, the issue of skills and resources can be addressed.

6. Answer: C
The client is motivated to pursue this avenue, and the OTA does not want to negate this motivation, even if the goal may be unrealistic. Begin with talking to the client to understand and support the motivation and follow up with formal or observational evaluation if necessary.

7. Answer: D
Hydration is especially important with seniors who may be on several medications and are always at risk of dehydration because of their age. The other issues are also important but can be addressed after hydration. Patients on some medications are especially at risk of sunburn.

8. Answer: D
Since vital signs (blood pressure, pulse, and respiration) are fine, answers A and B are not likely. It is possible to have migraine symptoms without having the painful headache, but this is extremely rare and not likely to only have fainting. Since fainting seems to be with movement, a vestibular disorder might be present and should be evaluated by an ear, nose, and throat physician.

9. Answer: A
A deadbolt should not be placed on the front door because a person with Alzheimer's could lock out the spouse when he or she steps outside for the newspaper or mail. The bathroom door lock should be removed so the patient does not lock out the spouse. The cellar door can be hidden with a sheet so the person does not try to open the door and gain access to dangerous supplies or tools. The stoppers should be removed to avoid flooding from forgetting to turn off the water. In addition, scatter rugs and stove knobs should be removed.

10. Answer: B

The managing OT should encourage the new OTA to present something she knows that the more experienced OTs and OTAs may not have learned in school. Changing the date involves another person and is not needed because the new OTA has the necessary skills to perform the inservice. Mosey's principles of teaching and learning that are basic to patient education can also be used for the new OTA in teaching and learning herself.

11. Answer: C

The garment is snug to prevent scarring but will not cut off blood circulation. Skin itchiness is often a complaint, and swelling or tenderness is sometimes a complaint.

12. Answer: A

The physician always makes the medical diagnosis; however, the OTA may provide some information concerning function related to the medical diagnosis made by the doctor. Answers B, C, and D, as well as pain management, joint protection, and environmental changes, are all part of work performance.

13. Answer: D

All the answers are of concern in eating/swallowing disorders, but the grading and altering of food size and texture may be the issue for this patient.

14. Answer: A

Forearm support may improve accuracy and will decrease fatigue and extraneous movements. Hand tremors may or may not be affected depending on the origin.

15. Answer: D

A person with aphasia may not be able to read directions; therefore, begin with a recipe known by heart.

16. Answer: B

Sitting while preparing food allows a one-handed cook the use of her knees to hold items. A home companion does not improve function. A photo cookbook is helpful for aphasia, and a forearm rest may help in feeding.

17. Answer: A

An angled foot stool reduces pressure on the back when sitting for long periods. A curved back chair with armrests helps the UE relax. A back support is for lifting and should be avoided by someone who sits all day.

18. Answer: A

Muscle strength is measured by MMT. Answers B and D also test strength but require more skill than MMT. ROM only tests the degree of movement; however, active movement against gravity assumes some muscle strength.

19. Answer: A

PROM done quickly through the available range usually assesses tone. A stretch reflex occurs if the muscle contracts. The OTA may not need to test for tone if the client can be observed in a flexor spastic pattern.

20. Answer: B

An arthritic person should open the jar using a rubber grip, turning away from disfiguring ulnar drift.

21. Answer: A

Co-contraction requires both extensor and flexor muscles to be active. This means the child must stay still, like in the game statue. Choices B, C, and D are activities that work on gross motor skills and require movement.

22. Answer: A

Subjective data is any data that the patient said. Objective data is fact-based from the OTA.

23. Answer: B

Job satisfaction is the number-one reason why staff stays in one facility. Salaries, benefits, and education, while important, fall below satisfaction.

24. Answer: C

Although great gains have been made lately, research in OT is still considered to be in its infancy when compared to other arts and sciences. Lack of research and evidence that OT works can lead to some people thinking of OT as a second-class science. For this reason, AOTF makes research a top priority.

25. Answer: B

A client with high distractibility requires an environment with low stimuli to focus on a task. Answers B and C are inappropriate. Answer D is not true.

26. Answer: A

Capital expenses are major costs such as land and buildings. Supplies and equipment are direct costs if used for treatment, indirect if used as office supplies. Staff salary is a direct cost of treating a patient unless the therapist is in a management position in which her management tasks are not billed to a patient and are considered an indirect cost.

27. Answer: D

Doorknobs should be located 36 inches from the floor to allow for access by a person using a wheelchair.

28. Answer: C

Documentation must comply with regulation and laws first. Management, OT staff, and, at times, faculty can provide suggestions within the regulations.

29. Answer: D

Only NBCOT offers certification for OTAs.

30. Answer: D

The patient needs to feel the value of a vertical position and to gain head control but still needs support in the wheelchair. If tipped back, she will never be upright; this does not treat the problem. Verbal commands will only lead to frustration of both patient and therapist. Using an object can help develop strength but cannot be used continuously.

31. Answer: C

Until you speak with the mother, you will not know the problem. The program may be too difficult, or the mother may be overwhelmed with the responsibility. When treating a child with severe disabilities, the OT is often treating the whole family. Take time to meet with the mother privately and provide her with the support she needs.

32. Answer: C

Persons functioning at cognitive level 5 (Allen) can make projects but are usually impulsive and disregard safety cues. Following a bus schedule would be too difficult, and making a sandwich would be too routine, although safety may be observed. A kit that snaps together likely has written directions that would be ignored. If a sample was available, this project could be successful but would not be the best project to challenge the client. The 1-day budget would begin to address the poor organization and would provide immediate feedback to the client.

33. Answer: B

The OTA must keep in mind the target audience when developing presentations. This audience would benefit from learning about the problems adults with mental illness face and how OT can address the weaknesses.

34. Answer: B

Medicare is for those aged 65 and over. Medicaid is a state health program for the poor. SSI/SSD is income for people over age 65 or people with disabilities. Welfare and Section 8 are state income programs for the poor.

35. Answer: D

Although documentation can help a health care professional in case there is an ethical claim, the purpose of documentation is to protect the consumer. Research, communication, and serial records are all benefits of proper documentation.

36. Answer: C

Playing dog involves extending the arms and head movement. Spinning on a scooter board is a vestibular activity. The balance beam activity may be too advanced for this child. Marbles are a fine motor activity.

37. Answer: C

The NBCOT exam can be taken only after all classwork and fieldwork are completed.

38. Answer: C

Vestibular stimulation has been correlated with an increase in verbalization, responsiveness, and muscle tone. Self-care may benefit if the child is directed to perform self-care activities. Behavioral modification techniques are helpful to address ADLs.

39. Answer: D

Too much vestibular input can cause emotional responses.

40. Answer: A

Problem-oriented medical record is a commonly used documentation system, especially in acute care facilities.

41. Answer: C

People with amputations spend more energy during ADLs than people without amputations. Adaptive equipment might help; however, energy conservation is first. Supervising others and cognitive retraining are only appropriate if there are deficiencies in these areas.

42. Answer: A

Although other areas of intervention would be valuable, working on integration of primitive reflexes will enhance overall development. Visual tracking and eye-hand coordination can be addressed after the reflexes. Small pegs are too difficult and dangerous for all 12-month-olds.

43. Answer: D

Expressive arts, such as art, dance, movement, and writing, are excellent resources to increase a patient's understanding of her dynamics and related feelings. Choices A, B, and C are task-oriented modalities.

44. Answer: A

Beneficence says that fees are fair and reasonable. Laws and regulations may also have been broken.

45. Answer: C

The first action is to speak to the therapist who made the comment. Although uncomfortable, as an occupational therapy practitioner it is your duty to stop an unethical practice. If the therapist continues with the plan to bill ahead, report the information to the Standards and Ethics Committee (SEC) of AOTA or other appropriate agencies. The SEC will provide you with information and support on how to handle the problem. Ethical problems are always difficult to address, but as an OTA, we have a high standard to protect our consumers.

46. Answer: D

A regular routine allows the greatest success in a bowel management program. Answers A, B, and C are standard practices for managing bowel programs.

47. Answer: C

Alcohol-free is the preferred pattern, but a minimum of 2 years is needed for maximum brain healing. Since alcohol may have been important to him prior to the car accident, may be the reason for the accident, and his friends reinforce the use of alcohol, the OTA must address this issue.

48. Answer: D

Lack of patient movement on a medical unit is more likely to affect patients with head injury, SCI, Guillain-Barré, and burns. People with multiple sclerosis are less likely to have heterotopic ossification.

49. Answer: A

Fatigue is the most common complaint as people develop stamina to gain independence. Depression and spasticity can be addressed with medication. Bladder control can be addressed with a regular schedule.

50. Answer: B

Some medications (Thorazine and some antibiotics) make people sunburn quickly. Sunscreen is extremely important. Clients may fatigue easily because of recent inactivity.

Section Four

1. Marketing occupational therapy services includes all of the following *except*:
   A. Needs assessment
   B. Environmental assessment
   C. Organizational assessment
   D. Market analysis

2. The OT in a small community program has been given permission to hire an OTA. During the interview process, the OT should ask the applicant all of the following *except*:
   A. Semi-structured, open questions asked of all applicants
   B. Personal characteristics
   C. Why he or she wants to leave the current job
   D. Job-related issues and characteristics

3. The following are contraindications for giving an elderly person a rocker knife *except*:
   A. Limited range of motion in the UE
   B. Tremors
   C. Cognitive impairments
   D. Lack of strong grip

4. What documentation procedure is likely to be challenged in a malpractice lawsuit?
   A. Patient response to evaluation
   B. Signatures that are legible
   C. Progress notes charted at the end of the day
   D. Records not fraudulently altered

5. Which approach is *least* effective in managing negative behaviors in brain injury rehabilitation?
   A. Work with the patient one-on-one in a quiet room
   B. Provide correct information when the patient does not know the information
   C. Expect the patient to participate in rehabilitation by allowing him or her to select simple, meaningful activities
   D. Use simple words and sentences, allow processing time, and repeat if necessary

6. An OTA is presenting a workshop at the local OT conference. The OTA wants to make copies of an article from the national association's journal to give to participants. What issue is *most* important?
   A. Copyright infringement; the OTA must have permission from the journal to make copies
   B. Copyright fair use; the OTA can make limited copies because it is a non-profit conference
   C. Copyright permission; the OTA can make unlimited copies because she is a member of the national association that publishes the journal
   D. Copyright registration; the OTA can check to see if the article is registered

7. Which is *most* effective in preventing contractures?
   A. Positioning
   B. Therapeutic exercise
   C. Serial casting
   D. Splinting

8. What is the focus of treatment for children with Rett syndrome?
   A. Increase tone
   B. Decrease stereotypical hand movements
   C. Decrease spasticity and ataxia
   D. Decrease rocking behaviors

9. What type of clothing do people with disabilities generally prefer?
   A. Slip-on type with no closures
   B. Fabrics that hold their shape and do not stretch
   C. Velcro closures on any type clothing
   D. Clothing based on their disability

10. What type of splint can control swan neck deformities and meet emotional issues?
    A. Small serial casting splint in bright thermoplastics
    B. Resting hand splint with Velcro closures in the color chosen by the client
    C. Silver ring splints
    D. Dynamic extension alignment splint

11. What handwriting tool would be *least* effective in a home program for elementary school-age children?
    A. Exercise putty
    B. Large slant board
    C. Assorted manipulatives
    D. Hair gel in a plastic zipper bag

12. Superficial heat agents are contraindicated for what condition?
    A. Stiff joints
    B. Muscle spasms
    C. Chronic arthritis
    D. Deep vein thrombophlebitis

13. What treatment option is *least* effective in controlling edema in a person with hemiplegia shoulder subluxation?
    A. Slings or shoulder taping
    B. Lapboard
    C. Arm trough
    D. Bilateral rolling platform walker

14. When is an OTA responsible for "duty to warn"?
    A. A patient is threatening bodily harm to another person
    B. An elderly person is being abused
    C. A child is being abused by an adult
    D. All of the above

15. What is the recommended slope for ramps added to an existing home to make it accessible to a person with a SCI?
    A. 6 inches of length for every 1 inch of height
    B. 12 inches of length for every 1 inch of height
    C. 18 inches of length for every 1 inch of height
    D. Whatever fits the property

16. All of the following supportive and compensatory strategies are effective in treating a person with low vision *except*:
    A. Eye patch
    B. Modify lighting
    C. Increase contrast
    D. Teach the use of visual markers

17. An effective fieldwork supervisor does all of the following *except*:
    A. Has a broad knowledge base
    B. Critiques constructively
    C. Has the supervisee figure it out on his or her own
    D. Takes the time to explain in the present

18. An OTA has recently been hired to replace an OTA who moved out of state. Management has asked for a QA report for the last 3 months. The former OTA never collected the data needed, and the data cannot be collected retrospectively. What should the OTA do *first*?
    A. Notify management that the data is not available and ask how the situation should be handled
    B. Notify management that the data is not available and present an alternative plan to retrospectively collect QA data
    C. Notify management that the data is not available and report the former OTA to appropriate state or national organizations for possible ethical violations
    D. Collect new data related to the current QA question and report that data to management

19. Intervention goals can include all of the following *except*:
    A. Occurrence of pain-free performance
    B. Gradation to more complex performance
    C. Improved quality of performance
    D. Assessment performance results

20. All of the following Standards of Practice can be done by both OTs and OTAs *except*:
    A. Educate referral sources about scope of services
    B. Follow defined protocols when standardized assessments are used
    C. Maintain or seek current information relevant to the client's needs
    D. Document recommendations for discharge follow-up or re-evaluation

21. The OTA shows a group of children several items on a table. While the children close their eyes, the OTA removes one item. The children open their eyes and guess which item is missing. Which of the following goals is *most* developed by the children?
    A. Increase eye-hand coordination
    B. Increase bilateral integration
    C. Increase form constancy
    D. Increase visual memory

22. Social smiling in infancy can be elicited by the mother at what age?
    A. 1 to 2 weeks
    B. 2 to 4 weeks
    C. 4 to 8 weeks
    D. 16 weeks

23. Universal precautions help prevent transmission of HIV and hepatitis B. The body fluids that universal precautions apply to include:
    A. Blood and other fluids containing blood
    B. Feces and urine
    C. Sweat
    D. Tears

24. A teenage girl with muscular dystrophy wants to apply her own make-up. As her OTA, you recommend all of the following *except*:
    A. Prop her elbow on the table to save energy
    B. Groom in phases with rest breaks
    C. Take a long shower before starting
    D. Enlarge the handles on the make-up items

25. A client who wants to use a computer but has only gross motor hand movement would use what type of input device?
    A. Standard keyboard
    B. Expanded keyboard
    C. Joystick
    D. Single switch

26. An outpatient client, 8 weeks postmyocardial infarction (MI), is tolerating walking 3 miles per day (2 mph) without pain. He has come in for a check of his rehabilitation level. While changing clothes, his wife mentions to the OTA that her husband is afraid to have sex because "he might die." What can the OTA tell this couple?
    A. Wait until he is more comfortable; this will likely happen in a few weeks
    B. Talk to his doctor for the approval; this is not to be decided by an OTA
    C. Refer the couple to the psychologist for further support
    D. Inform the couple that the MET level for sexual expression is the same as brisk walking

27. What food management issue is *most* important for a woman recovering from a right CVA with some left-sided neglect?
    A. Burning her left arm on the stove
    B. Dropping a glass bowl or knife and cutting herself
    C. Ignoring spoilage dates on food and becoming ill
    D. Forgetting items left in the oven

28. A person with shortened rhomboid muscles will not be able to:
    A. Comb the back of his hair
    B. Wash his LE
    C. Put a belt around his pants
    D. Brush his teeth

29. A male client is about to be discharged from rehabilitation services today at MET level 6 when the OTA asks if he has any further questions. He mentions, "Now that winter is on the way, how much snow can I shovel?"
    A. None until he talks to his doctor
    B. Light shoveling
    C. Shoveling (10 lbs)
    D. Heavy shoveling (14 lbs)

30. A client wearing a wrist splint has a reddened area that does not go away after 45 minutes. What should the OTA do?
    A. Add padding to the splint near the area causing the redness
    B. Adjust the splint near the area causing the redness
    C. Nothing special; this is not unexpected
    D. Have the client stop wearing the splint

31. COPD refers to all diseases that cause irreversible damage to the lungs. For a patient with COPD, all of the following activities are consistently difficult *except*:
    A. Decision making
    B. Eating
    C. Speaking
    D. Exercise

32. A young, healthy adult younger than age 40 will have blood pressure of less than:
    A. 120/80
    B. 130/90
    C. 140/80
    D. 140/90

33. A child must be able to identify body positioning in space and realize the course of movement to change his position to another position. This awareness of space direction will directly affect which of the following?
    A. Sorting one body part to another
    B. Reading and writing from left to right
    C. Picking an object out against a background
    D. Drawing a person

34. When speaking to a person with a hearing impairment, the OT should do all of the following *except*:
    A. Keep hands away from the face
    B. Speak slower
    C. Talk face-to-face
    D. Get the person's attention before starting to speak

35. How should flammable arts and craft supplies such as paint, stain, cleaners, and thinners be stored in the OT clinic?
    A. In a locked closet
    B. In an open area, supervised by staff
    C. In a ventilated, locked metal cabinet
    D. In a room with a sink and water

36. When a patient falls in the clinic, the *first* thing that should be done after ensuring the patient's safety and well-being is:
    A. File an incident report following the facility's policies
    B. Call the family and let them know
    C. Take the patient's temperature and blood pressure
    D. Notify the next shift of the problem

37. Prism glasses are ideal for:
    A. Patients with a halo or confined flat in bed
    B. Magnifying book pages
    C. Improving colors for low vision clients
    D. Not spilling drinks when patients have hand tremors

38. A child with spastic CP has scissors gait. This means the hip muscles are:
    A. In flexion
    B. In abduction
    C. Internally rotated
    D. Externally rotated

39. You are doing tactile and proprioceptive stimulation with a group of three children. The children are lying on a mat, and you are rolling a large ball over them. They like the feeling and ask you to do it again. What is the *best* response to the request?
    A. Say no; explain that they have had enough
    B. Repeat the activity, this time putting more pressure on the ball
    C. Say it's time to try something new
    D. Try bouncing the ball over them

40. Energy conservation techniques include all of the following *except*:
    A. Sit to work
    B. Limit amount of work
    C. Organize storage
    D. Plan 1 day at a time

41. Your 10-month-old client seems tired and frustrated during play activities designed to increase lung capacity. Although breathing appears normal, you check the child's pulse and find it is 120 beats per minute. What should be done *next*?

    A. Nothing; the pulse is normal, continue playing if the child cooperates

    B. Stop all activities and call a nurse

    C. Take a 5-minute rest

    D. End the treatment session early

42. There are numerous subtypes of personality disorders clustered into three groups of similar symptoms. Which cluster does *not* do well in occupational therapy group treatment?

    A. Cluster A—paranoid, schizoid, schizotypal

    B. Cluster B—histrionic, narcissistic, antisocial, borderline

    C. Cluster C—avoidant, dependent, obsessive-compulsive

    D. All clusters do not do well in group treatment

43. An adult with developmental disabilities is experiencing low vision problems affecting dressing. He is mismatching clothes and gaining attention at his grocery bagging job. All of the following are appropriate compensatory techniques *except*:

    A. Adjusting lighting in the closet or drawers

    B. Pinning or marking similar colored items to distinguish blue versus black

    C. Using large-print labels for organization on the closet doors

    D. Have caregivers match clothes in the closet on hangers

44. Brainstem sensations allow a person to get ready to do an activity. All of the following are associated with the brainstem *except*:

    A. Muscle tone

    B. Equilibrium

    C. Visual alertness

    D. Attention

45. An occupational therapy group for low functioning clients in a community setting focuses on self-management. What concept would be *least* effective to address this goal?

    A. Being on time

    B. Planning and making preparations on time

    C. Assuming responsibilities for errors and fixing them

    D. Expressing feelings of inadequacy

46. What is the *most* effective activity for assisting a young man with bipolar disorder to set self-limits when his attention span is less than 5 minutes?

    A. Creative painting to relaxing music

    B. Investigating heavy objects, such as a plaster sculpture

    C. Listening and clapping to songs

    D. Simple game, such as pencil toss

47. During an initial interview of hobbies, a person with schizophrenia tells the OTA that he has suicidal thoughts. What is the OTA's *first* response?
    A. Tell him that he is safe here in the facility, and the staff will help him get over these feelings
    B. Ask he if he has a suicide plan
    C. Tell him that this feeling is common in people with his disability and will get better with medication
    D. Notify the treatment team, specifically the doctor in charge of his care

48. What is the *best* occupational therapy intervention for a hospice family after their loved one has died?
    A. Help the bereaved family resume old roles and develop new roles
    B. Support the bereaved family by offering advice on getting over the sadness
    C. Leave the bereaved family alone to grieve in private
    D. Refer the bereaved family to support groups

49. What communication adaptation is *most* effective for decreasing confusion in middle stages of dementia?
    A. Large written signs posted in clear spots
    B. Give simple written instructions to the client to do simple tasks
    C. Use simple verbal commands, adding visual or tactile cues
    D. Teach the client that red signs mean no and green signs mean yes

50. What type of seating system provides the *best* pressure distribution?
    A. Linear
    B. Planar
    C. Contoured
    D. Generic

Section Four Answers and Explanations

1. Answer: A

Needs assessment is part of program development. Environmental assessment is examining the population served. Organizational assessment evaluates its effectiveness with the population. Market analysis is the use of information from the environmental and organizational assessments.

2. Answer: B

Personal questions are illegal. Only questions related to the job can be asked.

3. Answer: A

Limited ROM is an indicator for a rocker knife. All the other answers are safety concerns for a rocker knife.

4. Answer: C

Documentation principles include objective patient response to evaluation and treatment, follow-up instructions to family and friends, notations that are timely and legible, and records that are never tampered with. An attorney will question how a staff member could remember each patient's response after treating 8 to 10 different patients.

5. Answer: C

People with head injuries may not be able to make choices and may seem resistive to rehabilitation. A quiet, supportive, reassuring environment that can be processed by the person is most effective. As healing progresses, participation in the rehabilitation process will improve.

6. Answer: A

The OTA must request copyright permission to make copies from a journal or she is breaking copyright laws. Fair use is generally understood to be one copy for personal use. Registration is a moot point because any copies need the publisher's or author's permission. It should be noted that permission to copy is often very easy to get, especially for educational purposes. When the copies are to be sold for-profit, the copyright holder usually requires a small fee.

7. Answer: A

All the answers are effective treatments for contractures, including the addition of physical agent modalities. Once reduced, contractures can be avoided with correct positioning to encourage normalized tone.

8. Answer: B

Rett syndrome affects females beginning at age 8 months. Stereotypical hand movements include hand wringing, hand-to-head, and hand-to-mouth behaviors, leaving the child unable to play. Initially, hypotonia is present but later spasticity develops. The loss of purposeful hand movements limits the child's attention to play and leads to developmental issues. The hand movements are the focus of treatment.

9. Answer: A

A research study found that people with disabilities preferred clothes without closures that slipped on. Velcro-type fasteners were frustrating because they "looked disabled," felt rough, caught on clothes, and filled with lint. Participants reported they wanted soft clothes with stretch that made them feel warm. In general, they bought clothes for the same reason as nondisabled people, "to look good."

10. Answer: C

Silver ring splints are attractive jewelry that hold joints in extension. They can be worn on every finger. The other splints may be appropriate, but they look like medical devices.

11. Answer: B

All the tools are effective with the addition of squeeze toys and vibrating pens. A slant board might be used with some families, but it might not be practical for storage because of the size.

12. Answer: D

Superficial heat may be helpful for stiff joints, chronic arthritis, muscle spasms, and contractures but is contraindicated for DVT, tumors, impaired sensation, infections, and rheumatoid arthritis.

13. Answer: A

Taping or slings can control subluxation but do not assist in edema control because the hand remains in a lower position.

14. Answer: D

Although there are not any "all of the above" questions on the NBCOT exam, this answer is meant to educate the reader about the legal responsibility of duty to warn. Duty to warn means a practitioner must notify legal parties when a person or the public is at risk, even when it means breaking confidentiality. Each state and some local counties have their own rules, but abuse or bodily harm must be reported in all states.

15. Answer: B

Twelve inches in length for every inch in height is correct; however, outside ramps are longer (up to 20 inches) for every inch up.

16. Answer: A

Eye patching is a direct remediation for strabismic binocular vision disorders. Low vision does not respond to direct remediation. The other answers are effective compensatory interventions.

17. Answer: C

A good supervisor generates alternatives when the supervisee is struggling. This inspires confidence and trust in the relationship.

18. Answer: B

Notify management of the problem and possible plan. Next, the OTA should review state licensure laws and national organization code of ethics, and report any possible violations.

19. Answer: D

Assessment results are used to develop goals and are not reported in the goal section of documentation. Assessment results might be considered a baseline data set that could be integrated into goals. All the other answers are appropriate for intervention goals. Goals should be linked to Uniform Terminology. Further examples can be found in Moyer's 1999 *The Guide to Occupational Therapy Practice*.

20. Answer: D

The OT is responsible for this area. Both OTAs and OTs can complete the tasks in the other three answers. The *Standards of Practice* (AOTA, 1998) found in the *The Guide to Occupational Therapy Practice* (Moyers, 1999) can provide further information.

21. Answer: D

While other goals can be integrated, visual memory is primary to the game.

22. Answer: C

Social smiling occurs between 4 to 8 weeks. Infant smiles are endogenous and apparent in blind infants as well as sighted infants. Visual fixation occurs between 2 to 4 weeks. Spontaneous social smiling is evident at 16 weeks.

23. Answer: A

Universal precautions should be applied to blood and other fluids containing blood. Feces, urine, sweat, and tears have extremely low to non-existent rates of HIV infection unless they include blood; however, gloves should be used in cleaning any body wastes. Universal precautions include gloves, gowns, face guards, and cleaning with bleach and water. The therapist may choose to wear gloves when treating all patients to reduce spreading germs to the patient. Washing hands before and after all treatments is general good practice.

24. Answer: C
Taking a long shower before applying make-up may be too exhausting. Energy conservation is the priority for this teenager. Choices A, B, and D will all help conserve energy.

25. Answer: D
A single switch is for a person with only gross hand movements. Keyboards and joysticks require finger gross motor or some fine motor.

26. Answer: D
MET levels for brisk walking are the same as MET levels for sexual expression with a familiar partner. It is appropriate for an OTA who understands MET levels to share this information.

27. Answer: A
Left neglect, often seen in right strokes, puts the person at greater risk for burning the left arm and/or hand, as the person has limited feeling or cognitive awareness of the left arm. Answers B, C, and D might also be a risk but are not directly related to left neglect.

28. Answer: A
Shortened rhomboids will not allow for full shoulder flexion, so combing his hair will be difficult. The OTA will need to lengthen the muscle to achieve normal movement.

29. Answer: B
Light shoveling, gardening, skating, and fishing in waders are all 5 to 6 METs. Shoveling higher than light, as well as singles tennis and water skiing, are 6 to 7 METs. Heavy shoveling is equal to running at 8 to 9 METs.

30. Answer: B
Padding will only increase the pressure in the area. Answers C and D will negatively affect treatment.

31. Answer: A
Decision-making is difficult for a person with COPD only if the blood oxygen is decreased. Eating, speaking, and exercising are always difficult, if not impossible.

32. Answer: D
140/90 is normal for someone under 40 years old. 160/90 is considered normal if the person is over 40. Most doctors like to see blood pressure under these caps, and current research is exploring if these caps are too high.

33. Answer: B
A child's awareness of space and direction helps him to read left to right and place words on paper. Sorting and drawing represent body image, which begins in infancy. Picking objects out is an example of figure ground.

34. Answer: B
Speak at normal speed, tone, and volume. Keep hands away from your face, get the person's attention before starting, and talk face-to-face.

35. Answer: C
All flammable supplies should be kept in a ventilated, locked metal cabinet unless the label warns differently. Hazardous materials must be used and disposed of following strict regulations. Most facilities have a hazard waste management supervisor. Check with this person concerning supplies and consider non-toxic alternatives.

36. Answer: A
An incident report should be filled out immediately, while details are still fresh in the therapist's mind.

37. Answer: A
Prism glasses are eyeglasses that bend light 90 degrees, so a person lying on his or her back can watch television or read a book on their lap. Answers B, C, and D are not true.

38. Answer: C
Scissors gait means that the hip muscles are internally rotated, in extension, and adducted.

39. Answer: B
Repeating the activity with more pressure allows for gradual gradation of proprioceptive input and allows the children to control the activity. Bouncing the ball over the children is both unsafe and frightening.

40. Answer: D
Part of energy conservation is planning ahead to pace one's self and save energy.

41. Answer: A
Children from birth to 1 year old have normal pulse rates of 115 to 130. The childhood years are normal at 80 to 115. Adult years are 72 to 80, and later years are 60 to 72. Although the child may be tired, this is not a medical issue. Switch activities to something that may be more fun or reassuring to the child.

42. Answer: A
Cluster A does better with one-on-one treatment to establish trust with the practitioner. All other personalities do well, and groups are the preferred treatment for peer feedback.

43. Answer: C
An adult with developmental disabilities or mental retardation may not be able to read. All the other options should improve dressing.

44. Answer: C
Muscle tone, equilibrium reactions, physical sense of self, modulated arousal, and focused attention are brainstem activities. Vision is a cortex activity.

45. Answer: D
Inadequacy relates to self-worth. All the other answers relate to self-management.

46. Answer: B
All the activities are alerting to the CNS except investigating a heavy object, which is calming. A young person in a manic episode will need calming activities that can be adjusted to short attention spans.

47. Answer: B
Always follow up a statement about suicidal thoughts with probing questions about plans and activities. Although many people with mental health disorders have suicidal thoughts, as do elderly people and clients with physical disabilities, an OTA should investigate suicidal thoughts with all clients.

48. Answer: A
Although each family is different and has different needs, an occupational therapy practitioner's expertise is in roles. Generally, a practitioner should never give advice unless specifically requested, and even then the OTA should help the client come to his or her own plan. Answer B, "getting over" the sadness, is inappropriate because death is a sad event, and all humans have the right to be sad after a death. Support groups are acceptable for those who like groups, while private time to grieve is acceptable for those who prefer being alone.

49. Answer: C
Middle stages of dementia are marked with significant decreases in reading and writing. People at this stage are no longer able to learn new things. They may still recognize a stop sign but will not recognize that red as a color means stop.

50. Answer: C
A contoured seating system provides the best pressure relief. Linear and planar both mean flat seating. Generic can refer to several different seating systems, including contoured, but alone does not provide pressure relief.

Section Five

1. Assessment of client performance can be contaminated by the following:
   A. Infectious material at the test site
   B. The OTA cueing the client
   C. Hazards specifically added to the testing for evaluation
   D. The OTA following the standard administration

2. When assessing home safety, staging hazards in the home evaluation can provide effective feedback to the team, family, and client. The OTA must first use:
   A. Real hazards to simulate problems in the home
   B. Photos of hazards to have the client identify
   C. Judgment in deciding which hazards should be set up
   D. Cueing to the client

3. A person at the highest level of cognitive functioning following recovery from a head injury may still need some assistance to be modified independent in the following situation:
   A. Handling multiple tasks with breaks
   B. Completing familiar household tasks
   C. Keeping memory devices
   D. When sick, fatigued, or under stress

4. The *best* way to develop professional competencies throughout an OTA's career is:
   A. Attend conferences
   B. Return to school for more education
   C. Network with peers
   D. Develop a professional development plan

5. The *first* issue to be addressed in a community-based early intervention program for children with disabilities is:
   A. Play and play exploration
   B. Collaboration with family members
   C. Functional toileting
   D. Feeding

6. While doing a kitchen activity in a home evaluation, the client spills a glass of juice off the counter and begins to clean it up. What should the OTA do *next*?
   A. Stand by to grab the gait belt
   B. Tell the client to stop, the OTA will clean up the spill
   C. Have the client safely sit while the OTA cleans to the spill
   D. Move to a safer section of the kitchen until the spill can be cleaned

7. Concern over a unique clinical situation, the OT has completed an evidence-based practice research of the literature. The OT has reviewed the material and established a treatment plan with the OTA. What is the *next* step in the process?
   A. Discuss the research with the client in language free of professional jargon
   B. Notify the client of the treatment plan
   C. Gather the necessary supplies need for the treatment approach
   D. Notify the treatment team of the new approach

8. While recovering from an illness or accident, the client may also be recovering from:
   A. Loss of occupations resulting from the illness or accident
   B. Loss of income related to the illness or accident
   C. Medication side effects
   D. All the above

9. All of the following are primary areas of occupation for children in an early intervention setting *except*:
   A. Functional mobility
   B. Social participation
   C. Handwriting
   D. Toileting

10. An OTA is concerned about a client's driving skill and is questioning if a referral should be made to a driving specialist. *First*, the OTA should evaluate:
    A. Mobility alternatives such as public transportation
    B. Basic range of motion, vision, cognitive functioning
    C. The client's behind-the-wheel skills
    D. How open the client is to counseling

11. The *most* effective treatment for cumulative trauma disorders is:
    A. Rest from the activity that caused the problem
    B. Splints to immobilize
    C. Reduce edema
    D. Client education and activity modification

12. The Health Insurance Portability and Accountability Act of 1996 (HIPAA) covers the administration and fraud of insurance. This law requires practitioners have written permission from the patient before disclosing information of the following *except*:
    A. Providing treatment
    B. Obtaining payment
    C. Carrying out health care operations
    D. Talking with the potential patients

13. A mother of a child the OTA has been treating in a preschool program has become frustrated by her child's "escapes from the car seat" while she is driving. What is the *best* recommendation?
    A. Behavioral techniques applied each time the child gets out of the car restraint
    B. A car seat with better positioning and support
    C. A vest that fastens in the back and tethers to the seat belt
    D. A companion to sit with the child in the back seat

14. A client with a vestibular disorder is referred to the OT clinic for treatment. When the OTA greets her she immediately states, "The OT says you are going to make me dizzy as part of my treatment!" What would be the *best* approach?
    A. Reassure the client that she may be dizzy but will be safe
    B. Explain that dislodged otoliths are causing the dizziness
    C. State that many clients feel uneasy about moving and that this fear will be addressed before any treatment starts.
    D. Explain that activities will be graded before advancing to the next level.

15. Medications that might effect balance in clients include all of the following *except*:
    A. Anti-psychotic
    B. Anti-depressive
    C. Hypertension
    D. High cholesterol

16. A 4-year-old with developmental issues is working on developing finger control as a foundation to begin writing. The child enjoys active play independently but still has some behavioral issues that do not allow unsupervised play. All of the following fine motor activities would be good choices *except*:
    A. Putting coins in and out of a piggy bank
    B. Play dough art
    C. Paper airplanes
    D. Large refrigerator magnets

17. Brushing with a surgical brush is a treatment technique for over-responsiveness to sensory stimuli. This technique administers:
    A. Direct deep-touch pressure
    B. Light superficial-touch pressure
    C. Improved circulation to the skin
    D. Alternating alerting and calming responses

18. Elder abuse in an institution might be manifested by all of the following *except*:
    A. Lack of occupational therapy services
    B. Persons left unattended on the toilet
    C. Shortage of care staff on nights or weekends
    D. Bedsores on buttock, heels, or elbows

19. Appropriate environmental adaptations for visual impairments include all of the following *except*:
    A. Remove low coffee tables or magazine racks
    B. Place color tape on a cane to make it easy to find
    C. Mark stair treads with high contrast edges
    D. Improve lighting in common pathways

20. Work tolerance screenings can be completed after an applicant has been offered a conditional employment offer. During this screening, the occupational therapy practitioner can offer:
    A. A final employment offer
    B. Advise to the applicant about his job performance
    C. Reasonable accommodation options to complete the job
    D. A prediction of future effectiveness on the job

21. A functional reach screening shows the client is unable to move body parts independent of each other. The *next* area to screen is:
    A. Endurance
    B. Reflex testing
    C. Strength
    D. Postural control

22. A referral from a home care provider states concern for the client's cognitive and perceptual skills. A screening in this area includes all of the following *except*:

    A. Insight and awareness

    B. Orientation and attention

    C. Visual motor

    D. Neuromuscular endurance

23. A client having difficulty organizing and problem solving would benefit from further assessment of:

    A. Executive functioning

    B. Orientation

    C. Insight and judgment

    D. Affect and mood

24. A client would need to have what forward reach to access items on a standard kitchen counter?

    A. 12 inches

    B. 18 inches

    C. 21 inches

    D. 32 inches

25. What environmental adaptation would allow a wheelchair user to garden effectively?

    A. Watering wand to extend the hose

    B. Raised garden bed

    C. Extended reach garden tools

    D. Built up handle garden tools

26. During a home evaluation following sub-acute rehabilitation services for a CVA, the OT and OTA notice the client is unable to reach the toilet paper without balance issues. What is the *best* recommendation?

    A. Use a reacher already provided to the client

    B. Install grab bars for positioning on the toilet

    C. Substitute a freestanding toilet tissue holder that can be moved

    D. Install a commode near the bed

27. A client is experiencing sensory problems following a peripheral nerve injury that is interfering with his ability to return to work as an assembly line worker. He is receiving sensory reeducation as part of his therapy. What issue is addressed *last*?

    A. Hypersensitivity

    B. Scar tissue formation

    C. Strengthening

    D. Stereognosis

28. Which techniques could inhibit negative motor responses in a client with excess tone that limits participation in ADLs?

    A. Joint compression

    B. Icing

    C. Quick stretch

    D. Light moving touch

29. When positioning a client in bed lying on back, involved side, or uninvolved side using NDT principles to manage tone, which is *true*?
    A. Proximal musculature is positioned after the distal
    B. A head pillow is not used
    C. The head is supported with a pillow at midline
    D. Clients can maintain these positions for extended times because of pillow use

30. When training a client with unilateral neglect using visual scanning, which factor is *most* important?
    A. Visual preciseness
    B. Speed of eye movements
    C. Awareness of affected side
    D. Visual acuity

31. Which is *true* when adjusting a car seat for a child with a disability?
    A. Harness straps should have zero slack
    B. Head straps decrease the likelihood of injury
    C. Attached toys to the seat helps the child entertain him- or herself
    D. Padding can be added for additional support

32. All of the following are important concepts in pain management *except*:
    A. Clients learning to attend to the pain
    B. Relaxation techniques
    C. Increase physical activity
    D. Social support

33. Recline and tilt wheelchairs provide for all of the following *except*:
    A. Relief of pressure
    B. Posture management
    C. Added comfort
    D. Active mobility for low-level injuries

34. Under Medicare Part B rules group therapy rates must be charged if:
    A. The patient is seen individually but the family is present
    B. 2 clients are treated individually but at the same therapist's time
    C. The therapist is giving direct therapy services
    D. Any consultation services are provided

35. A home care client with diabetes begins to complain that he is not feeling well with sweating, shakiness, and fast pulse. The OTA stops treatment and
    A. Calls 911 as these are symptoms of a heart attack
    B. Makes arrangements for the next appointment when the client feels better
    C. Has the client test his blood sugar level and if under 110, have a snack
    D. Has the client test his blood sugar level and if under 70, have a snack

36. A client in treatment for breast cancer is experiencing the common side effects of chemotherapy including fatigue, loss of appetite, mouth sores, and common infections. She asks the OT and OTA to include complementary therapists in her approach to treatment. The OT and OTA agree and adds all of the following *except*:

    A. Focus on the complementary treatments that support long term goals in OT

    B. Documents intervention so client's progress can be measured

    C. Seeks additional information from magazines and health food experts

    D. Adds breathing, relaxation, guided imagery, aromatherapy, and massage to treatment

37. Occupations of a new born infant or premature baby in a neonatal intensive care unit include all of the following *except*:

    A. Sleeping

    B. Social interaction

    C. Procuring

    D. Feeding

38. What type of splint is preferred after trauma or surgery that involves an open wound?

    A. Commercial

    B. Modified prefabricated

    C. Precut

    D. Custom

39. Occupational therapy intervention for carpal tunnel syndrome includes all of the following *except*:

    A. Sensory and muscular assessment by the OT

    B. Electro diagnostics

    C. Functional loss evaluation by the OT or OTA

    D. Exercise and inflammation management

40. Sara Anne is an elderly woman living in a church elderly community that values conservative family values. Although she has elderly friends in the area she does not have any family except for sisters 150 miles away. The social worker is concerned that Sara Anne is at risk of a serious fall as she has had several "trips." The OTA servicing the population as an independent living counselor finds a woman that rarely leaves her apartment, is sometimes confused or dizzy, and reports being fatigued. What would be the OTA's NEXT approach?

    A. Refer her to her family medical doctor

    B. Address her fear of falling with counseling

    C. Educate her about home hazards

    D. Evaluate her ADLs

41. Diabetic retinopathy can cause loss of vision from retinal bleeding. Functional activities must consider all of the following *except*:

    A. Avoid heavy lifting

    B. Avoid bending head below heart level

    C. Avoid exercise and stretching

    D. Avoid holding breath or straining

42. Henry is an outpatient client with numerous medical conditions including post CVA, heart disease, long-term diabetes, low vision, and arthritis. He is a war veteran who took up smoking in the military service and has not stopped. He wears heavy eyeglasses and is unsure in his gait. He typically has a list of complaints when he arrives for his appointment. Counseling skills are appropriate intervention for all of the following complaints *except*:

    A. Stiffness in the morning when he wakes up

    B. Blurry vision and "things" floating in his vision

    C. Left hand weakness since his CVA

    D. Lack of friends since "they are all gone"

43. A client is referred to OT services for a functional assessment following a diagnosis of fibromyalgia syndrome. She reports both frustration and relief as it took 4 years for a "proper diagnosis." She has adjusted her life as she coped with "that unknown thing" but would like to sleep better so she has more energy during the day with her 4-year-old. The OTA helps the client establish sleep routines and habits by recommending all of the following *except*:

    A. Set aside some play time with the 4 year old each evening

    B. Limit activities in bed to sleeping and sex

    C. Add aerobic exercise each day

    D. Add strength training to the exercise routine

44. A client transferring from wheelchair to car seat has been successful in his training and is preparing to be discharged home when a new problem arises. Now that he is wearing his typical clothes he finds the corduroy pants he enjoys stick to the car seat fabric like burrs making transfers difficult. The OTA recommends:

    A. Continuing to wear the sweat pants he practiced in when in the car

    B. Switching to other clothes such as blue jeans

    C. Buying adaptive equipment to make the transfer easier

    D. Using a plastic garbage bag on the seat to ease turning

45. A recent immigration family has been referred to an outpatient clinic to address their daughter's preschool skills as she has spastic cerebral palsy. The parents were political refugees and are very happy to be in a new country, eager to help their children, but guarded about outside people. There are some language barriers and a translator is not always available. The mother states she wants her children to be successful in school and grow up "strong and independent." Range of motion is limited in the child's UE as the political nature of her parents forbid treatment in her former country. With hand use an important family goal, the OT recommends, serial inhibitory casting. The OTA is concerned that the casting might be worrisome to the family because its appearance of restraints, something the family has reported from their former country. All of the following is appropriate to educating the family about the option of casting *except*:

    A. Demonstrate on the child

    B. Write a description of the process and have a translator explain it to the family

    C. Have the family meet another family who is using this treatment method

    D. Use counseling techniques after explaining the process to the family

46. A child with spina bifida at the sacral level is being screen as part of the normal pre-registration process of entering kindergarten. The child had been seen by OTs and PTs in preschool programs but is currently not receiving services. The OTA expects to see what level of sensorimotor impairments?

    A. Variable weakness/loss from the waist down

    B. Paralysis of lower legs but some movement of hip and legs

    C. Weak foot flexion and some hip problems but other leg movements

    D. Mild weakness in lower leg

47. Social skills training is often used with people with serious and persistent mental health disorders. The OTA should use all of the following strategies *except*:

    A. Avoid feedback, allowing the client to self-evaluate performance

    B. Provide opportunities to practice skills in real life situations

    C. Use motivators and rewards that match the skills being taught

    D. Individualize education to the cognitive level of the client

48. While visiting a home care client for ADL training the OTA notices the client is unable to say no to telemarketers who call 3 times during the visit. All of the following are appropriate treatment approaches but which should be done *first*:

    A. Ask permission to put the client on the no-call national list

    B. Teach and practice assertiveness skills

    C. Role play how to handle telemarketing calls

    D. Report the problem to a supervisor

49. As the OTA providing services to a community living program that services the elderly with mental retardation, you have been asked to in-service the staff about hip precautions in preparation for the return of a resident who fell and broke his hip while gardening. Hip precautions include all of the following *except*:

    A. Crossing legs at ankles

    B. Crossing the legs at knees

    C. Hip flexion beyond 90 degrees

    D. Knee full extension

50. The OTA in the above situation is concerned that the resident will want to sleep on the unaffected hip because he likes facing the door in his bedroom and also watch his television this way. The OTA is concerned because:

    A. The affective hip will not have support in the bed

    B. The affective hip will be the lead extremity when raising out of the bed

    C. This encourages internal rotation of the affective hip

    D. This leaves the incision exposed

Section Five Answers and Explanations

1. Answer: B

A common problem in assessment is the OTA providing cues to the client. The practitioner must remember that assessment is not treatment and should follow the standard administration directions without providing assistance to the client.

2. Answer: C

Hazards can be excellent ways to assess a client's performance in their home however the OTA's judgment is most important.

3. Answer: D

A person at RLA level ten is able to complete A, B, and C without assistance but may become frustrated and irritable when tired or ill.

4. Answer: D

There are many ways to develop professional competencies including A, B, and C. A professional development plan is individualized map to achieving these skills. In addition, this plan assists the OTA in documenting skills to outside reviewers.

5. Answer: B

Collaboration with family will establish the occupations of the child and their current developmental level. The other answers may be appropriate following collaboration.

6. Answer: A

While safety is always first and the OTA must make a clinical judgment, this is a home evaluation and the client is likely to face this same situation without the OTA present.

7. Answer: A

The Evidence-based practice approach includes consulting with the client about what was found in the literature and how it might apply to the client. After agreement from all involved, the OTA would move forward to the treatment stage.

8. Answer: D

Although there are no "all the above" answers on the NBCOT exam, this question is designed to educate the reader to the multi-faceted nature of recovery.

9. Answer: C

Handwriting may be addressed as pre-handwriting skills however is typically addressed in the school system once the child has begun formal school. ADLs, play, and social participation are occupations of children from birth to three.

10. Answer: B

The other areas are also of concern to the OTA however a basic evaluation of performance would be helpful in establishing the next step in driving.

11. Answer: D

All the answers are appropriate treatment for cumulative trauma disorders as well as heat or ice however only D addresses the issue of reoccurring trauma.

12. Answer: D

HIPAA is a complicated law designed to protect patient's records. The administration of the facility has likely addressed this issue to assure timely payments from funding sources once treatment begins. An OTA can talk to potential clients about services available but would still be required to hold any information disclosed confidential under state laws and the AOTA code of ethics.

13. Answer: C

Although behavioral techniques might work, the mother may not be able to apply the techniques while driving. A car seat addressing positioning and support is best for the child with limited trunk control. A companion might be effective but may not be available. As safety is always the most important issue, the vest that closes in the back would be the safe option.

14. Answer: C

Clients with dizziness will be very guarded about moving and forming relationships with practitioners they think might make them dizzy. Although all the answers might be true, addressing the fear is the first issue. Answers B and D have professional jargon the person might not understand.

15. Answer: D

A, B, and C might have balance and falls as side effects of the medication. Statins, commonly used for cholesterol, are not known to cause problems with balance.

16. Answer: A

Although this is a fine motor activity, small coins or paper clips could be placed in the mouth and cause a safety issue. The other items might also be placed in the mouth but are bigger than coins.

17. Answer: A

This technique, know as the Wilbarger Protocol, uses deep pressure to calm over-responsiveness.

18. Answer: A

Although a facility would benefit by having OT services, this is not an automatic warning sign of possible abuse as may institutions service clients who might not benefit from direct services. All the other issues as well as poor hygiene, inadequate dental hygiene, unexplained weight loss, or person in soiled beds are signs of neglect.

19. Answer: B

Although an excellent treatment approach, marking a cane is adapting an assistive device. Environmental modifications include all of the other answers plus any task that alters the living situation.

20. Answer: C

The screener can offer accommodations to assess how the applicant performs the tasks of the job. A, B, and D should not be offered. A full ergonomic assessment by an OT might provide additional information and can be suggested in the screening process.

21. Answer: D

Postural control seems to be the issue related to the coordination of reach. The other areas should be assessed as well but an understanding of postural adaptation is the first issue to address.

22. Answer: D

Cognition and perception are interrelated processes required to see and use information in our daily lives. Endurance is a physical process that might effect cognitive functioning when low but is not part of the cognitive-perceptual assessment of a client. In addition to A, B, and C, visual processing, unilateral neglect, memory, and motor planning are assessed.

23. Answer: A

Organization and problem solving are upper level cognitive functioning skills. The ability to self-monitor is important to independence and should be further evaluated. The other areas mention might be appropriate to assess after executive functioning issues are addressed.

24. Answer: C

Standard kitchen counters are 21 inches deep, typically available to anyone who has full elbow extension and movement of the shoulder.

25. Answer: B

The other tools might be helpful but the gardener wants to be able to touch the plants from a sitting position.

26. Answer: C

The reacher might be helpful in the house but will not work with tissue. Grab bars might be a good idea for balance but the issue is likely reach. An inexpensive standing tissue holder will address this and not look like adaptive equipment in the bath.

27. Answer: D

Before Stereognosis can be addressed, especially for a worker who works on an assembly line; the other issues must be addressed. Strengthening might not be an issue.

28. Answer: A

Slow rocking or stroking, deep tendon pressure, and joint compression inhibit while the others facilitate motor response.

29. Answer: C

All others are false and can cause additional problems. Proximal motor control is addressed first to assist distal. The client's position must be moved a minimum of every 2 hours to avoid skin problems.

30. Answer: C

Lack of eye movements to the neglected side results in inattention.

31. Answer: A

Padding should never be added behind or under the child as this changes the straps' effectiveness. Head straps and attached toys increase the risk of injuries in an accident.

32. Answer: A

Cognitive restructuring and distraction are important aspects of pain management where a client learns to pull their attention away from the pain. Increase physical activity, relaxation, social support, stress management, and biofeedback are also helpful in the management of the pain.

33. Answer: D

Active users should have low back chairs for best mobility.

34. Answer: B

Group rates are charged when the OTA is seeing 2 individual patients at the same time.

35. Answer: D

If blood sugar levels are under 70, this likely explains the symptoms which should be addressed with 15 carbohydrates intake. This includes 4 oz fruit juice, sugared soda, or 8 oz low fat milk. The client should test his blood sugar again 15 minutes later and if normal, return to therapy. Heart attack is always a possible issue with people with diabetes as they have high risk factors. If you are unsure, consult the doctor in charge of his care.

36. Answer: C

Information from magazines, experts, health marketing tools are likely not evidence-based practice. The first rule of complementary therapists is first do no harm. The OT should use scientifically reviewed journal articles to research complementary therapies that are effective and share this information with the OTA.

37. Answer: A

Sleeping is a passive activity and not considered an occupation however getting ready to sleep is an occupation. Social interaction with family and staff, making needs known (procuring), and feeding are occupations of an infant.

38. Answer: D

A custom splint allows for adjustments to open wounds. Some commercially available products may allow some modifications however this varies.

39. Answer: B

Electro diagnostics is a medical test commonly done for carpal tunnel syndrome by the medical doctor. The other assessments are done by the OT/OTA team. Treatment may include exercises, inflammation management, and splinting with the goal of pain reduction.

40. Answer: A

Dizziness, confusion, and sleepiness might be due to medical conditions such as urinary track infections, postural hypotension, dehydration, or medicine side effects. All the other answers are also appropriate after all medical issues have been ruled out.

41. Answer: C

Exercise and stretching are healthy as long as within medical limitations. Consult the client's eye doctor or general physician for limits on lifting weight, blood pressure, or bending.

42: Answer: B

Immediately contact the client's eye doctor about a sudden onset of "floaters." As this client has diabetes, he may be experiencing a decline in his vision.

43. Answer: A

Play in the evening will likely get the child and mom in an alert stage that will make sleep for both difficult. Quiet routines and habits in the evening will assist in preparing for sleep. Exercise and strengthening are helpful in sleep if done earlier in the day. The bed should be used only for sleep or sex. Reading, eating, or playing should not be done in bed if the goal is sleep improvement.

44. Answer: D

This inexpensive and easily available tool allows the client to continue to wear his favorite clothes.

45 Answer: A

No casting should be done until the family and child understands the purpose and have discussed the issue of restraints especially since restraints are sometimes used as torture by some governments.

46. Answer: D

Answer A is Thoracic, L1, or L2. Answer B is L3. Answer C is L 4 or L5.

47. Answer: A

Persons with serious mental health disorders are likely to have weaknesses in insight and judgment making internal feedback inaccurate. The OTA should provide concrete feedback with specific examples of both positive and negative behaviors

48. Answer: A

The client may not know a no-call list is available but this still does not protect the client from some types of calls (charities and political). Teaching assertiveness skills is important but often difficult for the client to use initially. Practice of assertiveness skills adds to confidence. Discuss the issue with a supervisor, this situation may be financial elder abuse.

49. Answer: D

Knee extension is fine and used when the person must bend to pick something up. The effective hip is extended back, the knee is extended, and the unaffected hip is bent.

50. Answer: C

Internal rotation is not allowed in hip precautions. Placing the bed and television so the client does not roll on to his uninvolved side is important.

SECTION IV
Life After the Exam

Chapter Seven

Waiting for the Results

WAITING FOR THE RESULTS

Many OTA students have said to us that waiting for the exam results to be mailed back is almost as hard as studying for the exam itself. Generally, you can expect the results in approximately 3 weeks. Do not listen to rumors of how the results will look when you get them. I have heard that if the envelope says your name with OTA this means you passed. I have also heard that if the envelope is thick, you passed. These rumors are not true. The only way to know if you passed the exam is to open the envelope.

WHAT IF YOU DO NOT PASS?

Although the number of people who do not pass the exam to become OTAs is small (about 20%), the reality is that some students will not pass, and it may be you. There are many reasons why students do not pass the exam. When they took the exam, some had major stressors in their lives, such as a family illness or recent death. There are students who did well in school but may not be good test takers. Some students did not prepare for the exam by reviewing their weaker areas but simply reviewed their comfortable areas. Finally, there are those students who did not pass the exam for no clear-cut reason. Whatever the reason, it is my experience that you should not spend a lot of time ruminating over the fact that you did not pass. Of course, I realize that this is easy for me to say, and the bottom line is not passing the exam hurts a lot.

What To Do First

If you have accepted a job offer or have already begun working, you will have to notify your employer. If possible, speak to the director of occupational therapy. The director will understand more easily than non-occupational therapy staff, such as the personnel department. Depending on the licensure laws in your state, you may be able to keep your job working as an OT aide or rehabilitation associate while you study for the next exam. Keep in mind that you do not want to practice occupational therapy until you have passed the exam due to liability concerns.

Other than the licensing board in your state, who will receive your scores from NBCOT, no one else has access to your exam. This means that it is within your control to tell people that you did not pass the exam. I recommend that you share the information with those who can be supportive of you as you study for the next exam. It is important to know that your school does not know who did not pass the exam unless you tell them.

After you have notified your employer, you should check with the appropriate people for further information about working and studying. These people may include:

- the testing center for hand correcting the exam you took
- the program director at your school
- the state licensing board for occupational therapists for further questions
- your friends from school
- other OTs or OTAs who can help you study weak areas
- other professors whom you found helpful or supportive in school

Lastly, I would like to discuss the emotional aspects of not passing the exam. It is my experience that this is a strong factor on how students cope with studying for the next exam. Not passing the exam the first time around will seem like a major loss in your life. It is expected that you would deal with this loss in the same way that people usually deal with stressors. At first you can expect feelings of shock, anger, depression, and bargaining. Acceptance and coping will come later. Again, it is my experience that everyone does cope and is able to sit for the next exam. Generally, 2 months is enough time to develop coping skills. If coping is more difficult for you, seek professional help to deal with the stress. I believe that counseling or therapy is one of the best treats you can give yourself. Do not be afraid or feel guilty for seeking professional help. Your college counseling center can provide you with a list of local supports. There is a 90-day waiting period between tests.

How to Get Going Again

Keep in mind that you are not the only one who has not passed the exam this time. You are not the first one, nor will you be the last one. It is important to keep things in perspective to increase your ability to cope. The following is a letter from an OT who did not pass her exam on the first try.

To all students and future occupational therapy assistants:

At this point in my life, I think it is important for me to share my personal story with you. My teachers in college would have described me as an above average student, but I worked hard to be there. During my last affiliation, with much resistance and procrastination, I began to study for the OT boards. When the day arrived to take the exam, I was quite anxious. When I walked out, it was hard to know how I did, but I was confident I had passed. Ironically, I consoled a friend and classmate who was confident she had failed.

After waiting 4 long weeks, I received the results. I had FAILED. I kept staring at the words "you did not meet the requirements..." Not only that but there was an address to reapply.

I was supposed to be celebrating. They told us in school that "everyone passes" (or at least that was my perception). Despite many sad days and feeling unmotivated to try again, I got the books out and studied again. When I looked back, I realized that I had tended to study the information I knew and was comfortable with instead of focusing on my weak areas of practice.

This time I did my preparation differently. I studied in a group. I reviewed with peers. I used an outdated review book that provided me with structure. Lastly, I studied for many hours on my own. I focused only on my areas of weakness.

One thing that is important to mention is that I always had a tremendous amount of support from family and friends. With the support, the studying, and the courage to try again, I finally passed the exam the following year.

Although statistics show a low percentage rate for failing the exam, it does happen. It happened to me. My best advice is to not give up. Do your best and use supportive people to help you through the challenge. Although initially it was devastating, in the end it was a tremendous personal growth experience for me. I am currently practicing occupational therapy in an area that I enjoy, and I'm proud to be an OT.

My goal with this letter is to let everyone know that if you fail, you are not a failure. Do not give up even though you will have a strong desire to do so.

Best wishes to everyone,

J.T.

Making a New Plan

Once you are ready to start studying again, it is important to develop a personalized plan of action. Chapter Two of this book will take you through the planning process. For an OTA who has not passed the exam the first time, you may need some additional plans in place. Look carefully at what caused you difficulty the first time. Understand that you may never know for certain what went wrong on the first exam. Globally review all your class notes and focus on weak areas of practice.

Understand that periods of anxiety and sadness may creep back on you as you prepare to take the exam again. If you are a person who experiences test anxiety, taking the exam a second time will likely cause much stress. Consider a relaxation exercise, or visualize yourself calmly taking the exam and passing. Begin and end each study period with a visualization of you taking the exam and all the information you have studied flowing from your head, down your arm, and onto the exam. Feel yourself become calm, relaxed, and happy.

WHAT IF YOU DO NOT PASS AGAIN?

Should you not pass the exam for a second time, you need to know what options are available to you. We know some great practicing OTAs who have experienced this challenge. Again, do not give up. If in your heart you know that occupational therapy is for you, do a thorough self-assessment of what went wrong, seek the help you need, and prepare to take the exam again. NBCOT has recently lifted the three-test limit on taking the exam. In theory, a person has unlimited tries to pass the exam.

SUMMARY

Finding out that you did not pass the OTA exam will bring many emotional and cognitive challenges to you. Developing coping skills and preparing for the exam often will lead to passing the exam the next time. A thorough self-assessment of what went wrong the first time will help you develop an action plan. Notifying your employer if you are working and developing a support network of people who can help you study may be an effective way of coping with the challenges. Learning and using relaxation exercises may also be helpful. Whatever your options, do not give up; develop your resources, and use your supports.

Appendices

Appendix A

Selected Occupational Therapy Annotated Bibliography

The following books are suggested for study references when preparing for the occupational therapy assistant exam and were used by the authors as sources of information to develop content and domain-style study questions. I am thankful to these peers for developing such outstanding academic and scholarly works.

This list is a selected study reference list only. It would be impossible to list all the great occupational therapy books available. Endorsement is not to be construed, and the author recommends that students base his or her personal references on their coursework, as their faculty used a variety of textbooks to support their curriculum.

Allen, C. K., Earhart, C. A., & Blue, T. (1992). *Occupational therapy treatment goals for the physically and cognitively disabled*. Bethesda, MD: American Occupational Therapy Association.

Provides information on cognitive function, evaluation, and instruments using the cognitive disabilities frame of reference. Performance analysis is reviewed in detail, and treatment suggestions are provided.

American Occupational Therapy Association. (2002). *Official documents of the American Occupational Therapy Association. Bethesda, MD: Author.*

Extremely helpful official documents of the AOTA provide information on all aspects of occupational therapy practice.

Asher, I. E. (1996). *An annotated index of occupational therapy evaluation tools*. Bethesda, MD: American Occupational Therapy Association.

Provides an annotated list of over 100 assessments commonly used in occupational therapy. Each assessment includes target population, statistical information, and assessment sources.

Bonder, B. R. (2004). *Psychopathology and function* (3rd ed.). Thorofare, NJ: SLACK Incorporated.

Major psychiatric disorders are described according to symptoms, etiology, and prognosis with focus on treatment and function.

Bruce, M. A., & Borg, B. (2002). *Psychosocial occupational therapy: Frames of reference for intervention* (3rd ed.). Thorofare, NJ: SLACK Incorporated.

Six frames of reference in mental health are described in detail, including developmental, cognitive, cognitive-behavioral, object relations, behavioral, and occupational behavioral. Information on organic mental disorders and the suicidal patient is also included.

Case-Smith, J., Allen, A., & Pratt, P. (1996). *Occupational therapy for children*. St. Louis, MO: Mosby-Year Book.

Addresses common issues in development and conditions affecting children. Treatment aspects include developmental, physical, social, and emotional issues.

Chop, W., & Robnett, R. (1999). *Gerontology for the health care professional*. Philadelphia, PA: F. A. Davis.

Looks at aging from a biological, social, and illness perspective in a variety of health care specialties. Addresses reimbursement issues and financial problems of aging.

Christiansen, C. (2004). *Ways of living*. Bethesda, MD: American Occupational Therapy Association.

A detailed book that reviews social and physical ADLs from basic to community skills.

Christiansen, C., & Baum, C. (2005). *Occupational therapy: Performance, participation, and well-being*. Thorofare, NJ: SLACK Incorporated.

Provides a framework of occupational therapy and identifies links between theory and practice. Discusses reasoning and decision making necessary for competent practice.

Cole, M. (1998). *Group dynamics in occupational therapy: The theoretical basis and practice application of group treatment* (2nd ed.). Thorofare, NJ: SLACK Incorporated.

Provides a detailed and easy to follow seven-step group process. Discusses frames of reference and writing group protocols.

Crepeau, E. (2003). *Willard and Spackman's occupational therapy* (10th ed.). Philadelphia, PA: J. B. Lippincott.

A general resource for professional issues, including occupational therapy history, philosophy, occupational science, 11 frames of reference, Uniform Terminology, and practice issues across the life span.

Dunn, W. (2000). *Best practice occupational therapy: In community service with children and families*. Thorofare, NJ: SLACK Incorporated.

Reviews theoretical and evidence-based practice in family-centered pediatric practice from a variety of frames of reference.

Early, M. B. (1998). *Physical dysfunction practice skills for the occupational therapy assistant*. St. Louis, MO: Mosby-Year Book.

Similar in style to Pedretti, this text addresses acquired physical disabilities of adults.

Early, M. B. (2000). *Mental health concepts and techniques for the occupational therapy assistant*. Philadelphia, PA: Lippincott, Williams & Wilkins.

Addresses pathology and treatment aspects of mental health consumers with a focus on the role of the OTA.

Fiorentino, M. R. (1972). *Normal and abnormal development*. Springfield, IL: Charles C. Thomas Publishing.

An out-of-print classic that describes primitive reflexes on motor development in normal and abnormal children.

Gilfoyle, E., Grady, A., & Moore, J. (1990). *Children adapt: A theory of sensori-motor development* (2nd ed.). Thorofare, NJ: SLACK Incorporated.

Using spatiotemporal frame of reference, this text provides developmental-centered treatment approach to treating children. Developmental sequences are used to gain skill performance.

Hansen, R., & Atchison, B. (2000). *Conditions in occupational therapy: Effects on occupational performance.* Baltimore, MD: Williams & Wilkins.

Pathophysiology of major conditions most often seen in occupational therapy clinics is reviewed. Testing, medical management, and occupational performance are addressed in case study reviews.

Hemphill-Pearson, B. (1999). *Assessments in occupational therapy mental health: An integrative approach.* Thorofare, NJ: SLACK Incorporated.

Provides in-depth discussion on several commonly used psychiatric assessments, including independent living skills and work. In addition, a detailed chapter on the interview process is included.

Hinojosa, J., & Kramer, P. (1998). *Evaluation: Obtaining and interpreting data.* Bethesda, MD: American Occupational Therapy Association.

Evaluation and assessment basics such as psychometric standards and development are discussed. This book looks at standardized and nonstandardized assessments across the specialties.

Jacobs, K., & Jacobs, L. (2004). *Quick reference dictionary for occupational therapy* (4th ed.). Thorofare, NJ: SLACK Incorporated.

Provides definitions of occupational therapy terms, concepts, and conditions with informative appendices.

Jacobs, K., & Logigian, M. (1999). *Functions of a manager in occupational therapy* (3rd ed.). Thorofare, NJ: SLACK Incorporated.

This text covers a wide variety of management and administrative responsibilities in occupational therapy.

Kaplan, H. I., Sadock, B. J., & Grebb, J. A. (2002). *Synopsis of psychiatry.* Baltimore, MD: Williams & Wilkins.

An extensive reference and explanation of DSM-IV TR, including all psychiatric classifications from a variety of theoretical models. Clinical explanations and classic treatments are described in detail.

Kaplan, K. L. (1988). *Directive group therapy.* Thorofare, NJ: SLACK Incorporated.

Provides concepts and practical guidance to this practice model designed specifically for the person functioning at a minimal level.

Katz, N. (1998). *Cognition and occupation in rehabilitation.* Bethesda, MD: American Occupational Therapy Association.

Complete coverage of a variety of cognitive issues across the specialties, including mental health and traumatic brain injury.

Kiernat, J. (1991). *Occupational therapy and the older adult: A clinical manual.* Gaithersburg, MD: Aspen.

Reviews aging, functional changes, and adaptation of adults over 65 years. Treatment information includes the role of fitness, empowerment, preventing falls, and cognitive aspects. Medicare is fully reviewed. Both community and long-term treatment are discussed in detail, including assessment, treatment, and discharge planning.

Law, M. (1998). *Client-centered occupational therapy.* Thorofare, NJ: SLACK Incorporated.

Explains the models available to center treatment around the client's goals. The Canadian Model of Occupational Performance (CMOP) is fully explained.

Levangie, P. (2001). *Joint structure and function: A comprehensive analysis.* Philadelphia, PA: F. A. Davis Company.

Basic theory of joint structure and muscle action necessary to understanding both normal and abnormal function. A review of biomechanics is included.

Lohman, H., Padilla, R., & Byers-Connon, S. (1997). *Occupational therapy with elders: Strategies for the COTA.* St. Louis, MO: Mosby-Year Book.

Holistically addresses issues of aging and the common problems with treatment focus.

Moyers, P. (1999). The guide to occupational therapy practice. Bethesda, MD: American Occupational Therapy Association.

A comprehensive review of the literature that supports the field of occupational therapy. Basic concepts, such as the OT process and referrals, are addressed. Excellent when explaining occupational therapy to another profession.

National Board for Certification in Occupational Therapy. (Spring, 2004). *Report to the profession*. Gaithersburg, MD; Author.

Reed, K. L. (2003). *Quick reference to occupational therapy*. Gaithersburg, MD: Aspen.

An excellent review of common disorders across the age span and disability practice. Information on cause, assessment, and treatment is provided in outline format. Precautions and outcomes are described. References and further readings specific to each disorder are provided.

Ryan, S., & Sladyk, K. (2001). *Ryan's occupational therapy assistant: Principles, practice issues, and techniques* (3rd ed.). Thorofare, NJ: SLACK Incorporated.

An overview of occupational therapy assistant practice including history, philosophy, Uniform Terminology, activity analysis, practice issues across the age and disability span, treatment techniques, and management issues.

Sladyk, K. (1997). *OT student primer: A guide to college success*. Thorofare, NJ: SLACK Incorporated.

Basic occupational therapy concepts and techniques are reviewed. Tutorials are provided as well as advice on managing learning occupational therapy.

Sladyk, K. (2003). *OT study cards in a box*. Thorofare, NJ: SLACK Incorporated.

A deck of index-sized cards review the major content areas for fieldwork, NBCOT exam, and practice. An OTA set is also available.

Trombly, C., & Radomski, M. (2002). *Occupational therapy for physical dysfunction*. Baltimore, MD: Williams & Wilkins.

Principles of practice in adult physical dysfunction are featured. Major diagnosis areas are addressed with focus on assessment and treatment. Numerous photographs illustrate basic techniques.

Wilcock, A. (1998). *An occupational perspective of health*. Thorofare, NJ: SLACK Incorporated.

Examines the relationship of health and occupation by defining and exploring occupation biologically and socially.

Williams, L., Pedretti, L., & Early, M. B. (2001). *Occupational therapy skills for physical dysfunction*. St. Louis, MO: Mosby.

A basic reference for clinicians, this text provides the application techniques for the treatment of adults with acquired physical dysfunction. Evaluation and treatment issues are completely addressed.

Zemke, R., & Clark, F. (1996). *Occupational science: The evolving discipline*. Philadelphia, PA: F. A. Davis.

Provides a model for understanding occupation as a science and art before examining occupational therapy treatment as an end means.

Zoltan, B. (1996). *Vision, perception, and cognition: A manual for the evaluation and treatment of the neurologically impaired adult* (3rd ed.). Thorofare, NJ: SLACK Incorporated.

Defines and outlines the theoretical basis of visual, perceptual, and cognitive deficits. Evaluation procedures and treatment are also identified.

www.nbcot.org—NBCOT's website provides up to the moment current information about the exam. Students should check the Web site at least monthly during their last year in school.

Appendix B
Common Abbreviations

The following is a list of abbreviations you may find helpful. You do not need to commit them to memory for the OTA exam; however, a working knowledge is useful.

AAROM	Active Assistive Range of Motion
ADA	Americans with Disabilities Act
ADL	Activities of Daily Living (or ADLs not ADL's)
AIDS	Acquired Immune Deficiency Syndrome
AOTA	American Occupational Therapy Association
AOTF	American Occupational Therapy Foundation
AROM	Active Range of Motion
CARF	Commission of Accredited Rehabilitation Facilities
COPD	Chronic Obstructive Pulmonary Disease
COTA	Certified Occupational Therapy Assistant
CVA	Cerebral Vascular Accident
DIP	Distal Interphalangeal
DRG	Diagnostic-Related Groups
FOR	Frame of Reference
HMO	Health Maintenance Organization
JCAHO	Joint Commission of Accreditation of Healthcare Organizations
MCP	Metacarpal Phalangeal

MET	Metabolic Equivalents Test
MMT	Manual Muscle Test
MORE	Measurable, Observable, Realistic, Explicit
NBCOT	National Board for Certification of Occupational Therapy
NSAIDs	Non-Steroidal Anti-inflammatory Drugs
OBRA	Omnibus Budget Reconciliation Act
OSHA	Occupational Safety and Health Administration
OT	Occupational Therapy, Occupational Therapist
OTR	Occupational Therapist, Registered
PIP	Proximal Interphalangeal
POMR	Problem-Oriented Medical Record
PRN	Whenever Necessary, As Needed
PROM	Passive Range of Motion
ROM	Range of Motion
SOAP	Subjective, Objective, Assessment, Plan
SSI/SSD	Social Security Insurance/Social Security Disability

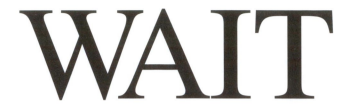

WAIT

...There's More!

Ryan's Occupational Therapy Assistant: Principles, Practice Issues and Techniques, Third Edition
Sally E. Ryan, COTA, ROH, Retired and Karen Sladyk, PhD, OTR/L, FAOTA
528 pp., Soft Cover, 2001, ISBN 1-55642-407-8,
Order #34078, **$55.95**

The reformulation of *Ryan's Occupational Therapy Assistant: Principles, Practice Issues and Techniques, Third Edition* includes occupation-based case studies that highlight the didactic material presented in each chapter, along with an updated style of information. With this clearly written third edition, the authors provide information in a student-friendly manner.

Quick Reference Dictionary for Occupational Therapy, Fourth Edition
Karen Jacobs, EdD, OTR/L, CPE, FAOTA and Laela Jacobs, OTR
600 pp., Soft Cover, 2004, ISBN 1-55642-656-9,
Order #36569, **$26.95**

This definitive companion provides quick access to words, their definitions, and important resources used in everyday practice and the classroom. Used by thousands of your peers and colleagues, the *Quick Reference Dictionary for Occupational Therapy, Fourth Edition* is one of a kind and needed by all in the profession.

Foundations of Pediatric Practice for the Occupational Therapy Assistant
Amy Wagenfeld, PhD, OTR/L and Jennifer Kaldenberg, MSA, OTR/L
432 pp., Soft Cover, 2005, ISBN 1-55642-629-1,
Order #36291, **$38.95**

Management Skills for the Occupational Therapy Assistant
Amy Solomon, OTR and Karen Jacobs, EdD, OTR/L, CPE, FAOTA
176 pp., Soft Cover, 2003, ISBN 1-55642-538-4,
Order #35384, **$30.95**

OT Study Cards in a Box, Second Edition
Karen Sladyk, PhD, OTR/L, FAOTA
255 Cards with Carrier, 2003, ISBN 1-55642-620-8,
Order #36208, **$43.95**

OT Student Primer: A Guide to College Success
Karen Sladyk, PhD, OTR/L, FAOTA
348 pp., Soft Cover, 1997, ISBN 1-55642-318-7,
Order #33187, **$32.95**

The Successful Occupational Therapy Fieldwork Student
Karen Sladyk, PhD, OTR/L, FAOTA
240 pp., Soft Cover, 2002, ISBN 1-55642-562-7,
Order #35627, **$35.95**

Ordinary Miracles: True Stories About Overcoming Obstacles & Surviving Catastrophes
Deborah R. Labovitz, PhD, OTR/L, FAOTA
416 pp., Soft Cover, 2003, ISBN 1-55642-571-6,
Order #35716, **$16.95**

Documentation Manual for Writing SOAP Notes in Occupational Therapy
Sherry Borcherding, MA, OTR/L
256 pp., Soft Cover, 2000, ISBN 1-55642-441-8,
Order #34418, **$29.95**

Vision, Perception, and Cognition: A Manual for the Evaluation and Treatment of the Neurologically Impaired Adult, Third Edition
Barbara Zoltan, MA, OTR
232 pp., Soft Cover, 1996, ISBN 1-55642-265-2,
Order #32652, **$33.95**

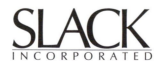